The Official Training Manual

TRANSFORMING
THERAPY

*A New Approach
to
Hypnotherapy
by*

GIL BOYNE

Hypnotherapy in the United States

The Genesis of Transforming Therapy

Transforming Therapy at Work

The Techniques of Transforming Therapy

WESTWOOD PUBLISHING COMPANY, INC.
GLENDALE, CALIFORNIA

Published by

Westwood Publishing Company, Inc.

700 S. Central Ave., Glendale, CA 91204

Telephone (818) 242-1159

In certain case histories contained herein, some names have been changed.

ISBN 0-930298-13-6

Printed in the United States of America

To my wife, Andreina, for her loving support

To my daughter Colleen for the joy of her childhood
and the bright promise of her maturity

To my son, Neal, for following his dream

To my mother for her love of the blues

To my father for instilling in me the work ethic

and

To Dr. Frederick Perls, whose teaching transformed my career

and finally,

I thank God that I was born in the United States of America
where each of us is free to create our own visions
and pursue our dreams

Other Works by Gil Boyne

How to Hypnotize: A Learning Guide
Marketing Self-Hypnosis and Other Group Programs

CONTENTS

Author's Preface   vii

Hypnotism: Key to the Creative Mind   ix

The Short-Term Hypnotherapy of Gil Boyne   xi

An Introduction to Transforming Therapy   xiii

Part One: The Genesis of Transforming Therapy

The Legal Basis for *Hypnotherapist*   3

Recognition for Hypnotherapy Training Programs   5

Transforming Therapy: A New Approach to Hypnotherapy   7

Hypnotherapy vs. Psychotherapy:
   Is There a Real Difference?   10

Part Two: Transforming Therapy at Work

Hypnotherapy to Overcome Mental Blocks
   The Case of Scotty ("The World's Worst Speller")   15

Hypnotherapy for Overcoming Performance Anxiety
   The Case of Pat ("Fear of Public Speaking")   97

Hypnotherapy to Stop Projection of Childhood Fears
   The Case of Holly ("You Scare Me")   109

Hypnotherapy to Change Lifestyles
   The Case of Nancy ("You Make Me So Mad")   125

Hypnotherapy to Find Lost Objects
   The Case of Claudia ("The Lost Diamond Necklace")   155

Hypnotherapy to Develop Self-Esteem and to Overcome
Alcoholism

    The Case of Bud ("Born to Lose")   187

Hypnotherapy to Cure Impotence

    The Case of Tyler ("I Can't Get It Up at the
    Right Time")   243

Hypnotherapy to Cure Stuttering

    The Case of Leo the San Diego Stutterer
    ("Please Don't Cut It Off!")   303

Part Three: The Techniques of Transforming Therapy

Pre-Induction, Goal Setting, Uncovering
Techniques, and Age Regression   351

Specific Techniques Used to Elicit Information   354

Reeducation and Reprogramming   357

Gestalt Dialogues   361

Pre-Trance Termination   367

Post-Trance Termination   367

Other Useful Ideas and Concepts   372

The "Experts" Attempt to Define *Hypnosis*   379

Experts Address the Safety of Hypnosis   382

Index   385

AUTHOR'S PREFACE

This book is addressed primarily to the student, the teacher, and the practitioner of hypnotherapy.

The case histories are exact transcripts from live therapies on videotape, not disguised reconstructions from notes or memory.

Whenever possible, I have avoided psychoanalytic terminology so as to make the work easily understandable and useful. I have shown the significance of specific methodologies in the context of my clinical work.

A major purpose of this work is to illustrate how a comprehensive theory of hypnotherapy can be formulated and utilized in an effective and practical way. My therapeutic choices and interventions are an expression of the underlying principles of transformation.

What I have written is in no way intended to be final or complete, but is designed to serve as another step forward in the rapid and continuing development that hypnotherapy is experiencing.

HYPNOTISM: KEY TO THE CREATIVE MIND

From the *Introduction* to *Practical Lessons in Hypnotism, by William Wesley Cook, M.D., 1901*

Hypnotism is the most practical science of the age. It enters into our everyday life, and confers advantages that cannot be acquired through any other medium. Its practice is no longer a mere pastime for amusement and sensation: as professional practitioners of the highest standing now recognize its value and seek to profit by its benefits. Scientists regard it as a natural power, for ages kept dormant, but apparently destined to perform an active part in the welfare and development of future generations.

To study hypnotism is to fathom the hidden mysteries of magic and human miracles and making them matters of absolute knowledge. Its possibilities are almost boundless and are interwoven with every phase of human life, and its powers are largely responsible for the successful terminations of modern business and social undertakings.

It does not require years of study to become a hypnotist, for this great blessing to mankind is a natural endowment possessed by practically everyone and capable of being developed by all who will devote to its study the patience and energy always so necessary for the development of natural talents.

The reward is great that follows the persistent study of hypnotism: for it is a science that bestows upon its devotees a power that seems almost superhuman. It overawes everyone who witnesses its indisputable facts and its marvelous manifestations. It overthrows the theories of judges and philosophers and theologians, and shakes the faith of material scientists in their preconceived opinions. It supplants the physician and the surgeon and cures the afflicted and deformed whom they pronounced beyond the hope of recovery. It breaks the chains of demoralizing and destructive habits. It comforts the sorrowing and brings peace of mind to those distracted by the perplexities of life. It abolishes periods of time and extents of distance. It causes the lame to walk and strengthens the weak. It checks the hand of death and snatches almost from the grave the grim destroyer's victims. It loosens the tongue of the stammerer, overcomes the self-consciousness of the socially shy and tempers the impetuosity of the rash enthusiast. To mankind, in every walk of life, hypnotism is a blessing—leading his innermost thoughts to higher and nobler things: developing his powers to plan and to execute and giving him social, financial and intellectual eminence among his fellowmen. All this, and more is Hypnotism.

THE SHORT-TERM HYPNOTHERAPY OF GIL BOYNE

Numerous books have been written about the unusual and innovative methods of Dr. Milton Erickson, but until now, none have been written about the amazingly rapid and successful methods of Gil Boyne. Erickson was a creative genius who devised many unusual and beneficial therapy methods. Gil Boyne is the genius of short-term, result-oriented therapy.

In his training programs, Gil Boyne repeatedly demonstrates that it is possible to transform the lives of people who have been programmed for failure, frustration, and unhappiness.

His personal fascination with transforming energy goes far beyond teaching. He leads people into that energy so that they can experience it in themselves.

He teaches that doing therapy is primarily an art form. He has an uncanny skill in making immediate contact with people therapeutically. He insists upon the client taking full responsibility for his present state of affairs.

When Boyne is engaged in his work, he is exquisitely sensitive and yet he maintains an incredibly relaxed manner. His genius as a therapist is his improvisational creativity.

He acts as a catalyst bringing people into a more clear state. He sees what they need, and he seems to produce changes magically.

Neophyte and veteran hypnotherapists alike report that his teachings not only alter their way of doing therapy but transform their personal lives as well.

Boyne feels that most psychotherapy is interminable and that treatment doesn't have to be prolonged indefinitely. His major principle is that you can always go towards health. He teaches about an "inner grace" that we can connect with and that hypnotherapy is always directed toward health. He starts with the premise that wholeness is the goal and we can go to wholeness because we have all the ingredients. We don't have to "get rid of" anything! Instead, we transform and add so that a whole person is created. Hypnotherapy is a hopeful work; psychoanalysis is always pessimistic. "Hypnotherapy," he says, "is not like surgery or medicine. It's not just techniques that can be taught. To be a good hypnotherapist, a person has to have an instinct for it—an inherent kindness and an ancient wisdom."

You, too, can change fragmented, unhappy people into integrated, happy people when you make use of Gil Boyne's principles of Transforming Therapy.

Adapted from *Miracles On Demand*, First Edition

AN INTRODUCTION TO TRANSFORMING THERAPY

Modern hypnotherapy has become the most dramatically effective short-term therapy developed to date. However, unlike many other modalities, it is very difficult to get comprehensive training in hypnotherapy today. It is rare to find even brief and limited courses offered in medical schools or graduate schools of psychology.

Life experience, personal therapy, and the influence of a memorable instructor are the primary forces that shape the hypnotherapist's career, yet there are very few competent instructors in this field. Medical schools and university graduate schools rarely have a faculty member qualified to offer hypnotherapy training. Psychoanalysts still voice objections to hypnotherapy based on theoretical positions formulated by Sigmund Freud near the turn of the century. Only a handful of mental health professionals have developed the special skills and cultivated the art of effective hypnotherapy practice.

As a practitioner and teacher of hypnotherapy for almost forty years, I have devised a highly specialized and carefully structured system of training. Lectures, demonstrations, and "feedback discussions" are combined with supervised practice sessions which initiate the student into the diverse aspects of trance training and behavior change.

Lessons quickly change from simple to complex. Theories are simplified and kept to a minimum, and the emphasis is always on producing therapeutic change and stimulating transformation.

Live therapies are videotaped and later presented on state-of-the-art projection equipment in larger-than-life images. Audio tapes and videotapes, training manuals, and textbooks are provided for students' continuing home study.

Transforming Therapy contains the actual word-for-word transcripts of videotaped therapy sessions. Participants are not actors demonstrating therapy techniques, but are actual therapy clients presenting real-life problems.

In most cases, these are short-term therapies with rapid and dramatic closures and solutions. In appropriate cases, long-range follow-ups are included. The result is a structural outline of each step involved as well as the actual wording used in procedures such as age regression, cathartic abreaction, gestalt dialogues, reeducation and repro-gramming, establishing trust, intensifying the underlying feeling, dis-covering the initial sensitizing event, and many other uncovering and processing techniques that are integral parts of Transforming Therapy.

Part One

The Background of Hypnotherapy as Practiced Today in the United States:

The Genesis of "Transforming Therapy"

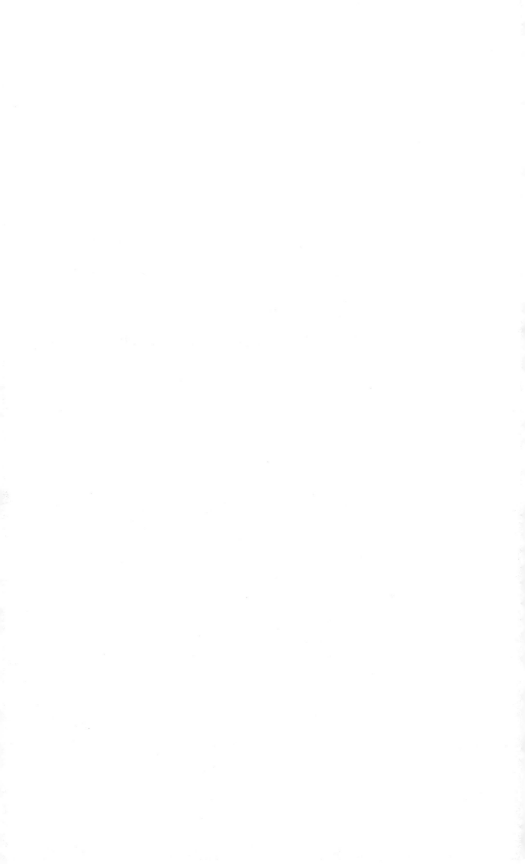

THE LEGAL BASIS FOR *HYPNOTHERAPIST*:
A BRIEF HISTORY

079.157.010 – Hypnotherapist
As defined in the Dictionary of Occupational Titles
Published by the United States Department of Labor

> "Hypnotherapist induces hypnotic state in client to increase motivation or alter behavior pattern through hypnosis. Consults with client to determine the nature of problem. Prepares client to enter hypnotic states by explaining how hypnosis works and what client will experience. Tests subjects to determine degrees of physical and emotional suggestibility. Induces hypnotic techniques of hypnosis based on interpretation of test results and analysis of client's problem. May train client in self-hypnosis conditioning."

The *Dictionary of Occupational Titles* (*D.O.T.*) is a reference manual published by the U.S. Department of Labor.

The book is compiled by input from many sources. One of the primary sources is the local Employment Development Center office in Los Angeles. The *D.O.T.* assigns numbers to and defines occupations. The U.S. Department of Labor is not concerned with what is or is not a state-licensed occupation, only that it is a legally and widely accepted occupation. Employment Development, Insurance, and many other departments of both the national and state governments use the book.

D.O.T. *Adds "Hypnotherapist"*

In 1975, as a result of the efforts of hypnotherapists Gil Boyne and John Kappas, the Department of Employment defined "Hypnotherapist" and an identification number was assigned (079.157.010).

In early 1977, the *Dictionary of Occupational Titles* appeared with the definition shown on page 3. This was the first formal recognition and identification of hypnotherapy as a defined occupation.

Definition Non-Medical

You will notice that the definition contains no medical terms, nor does it say you have to be licensed as a physician, psychologist, or social worker. It simply means that the U.S. Department of Labor defines *hypnotherapist* in the specific ways stated.

Not a Licensed Profession

As of this writing, there never has been a formal opinion in any of the United States of America that the occupational title "Hypnotherapist" is restricted to those holding a license in the healing arts or counseling professions.

In 1971, California Senator James Whetmore asked the question, "Is the practice of hypnotism restricted by state law to persons licensed to practice medicine or psychology?" The answer came in the form of a formal ruling from the California Attorney General:

> OPINION #17-24-April 14, 1971. "The practice of hypnotism is not prohibited by state law unless such practice constitutes the unauthorized practice of medicine or psychology."

You have a constitutionally guaranteed civil right to pursue gainful employment in a lawful (not forbidden by law) occupation. Don't be misled by those who fail to understand the law. Legislative committees in numerous states have repeatedly determined that licensing of an occupational group shall be required only when the unlicensed practice is proven to represent a threat to public health and safety. There has never been a documented case of harm from the use of hypnosis. Therefore, hypnotherapy remains a non-licensed profession!

RECOGNITION FOR HYPNOTHERAPY TRAINING PROGRAMS

On April 5, 1989, Gil Boyne presented the following program description to the Classification of Instructional Programs (CIP) Review Meeting, U.S. Department of Education, Office of Educational Research and Improvement, Washington, D.C.

Program Description: Hypnotherapy Training

"An instructional program that prepares individuals to use hypnosis (trance) as the primary technique in a process of reeducation at the mental/emotional levels for the purposes of solving problems, developing motivation, and setting and achieving goals. Teaches applications of hypnosis in health sciences and human services. Prepares students for certification examination."

It was accepted and approved by the National Center for Educational Statistics, U.S. Department of Education, on April 7, 1989, for inclusion in *A Classification of Instructional Programs*, published by the U.S. Department of Education every five years.

Hypnotherapy Training Program has been assigned a six-digit identification number and is classified under "Human Services" in the "Health Sciences and Human Services" division.

This is the first formal recognition and identification of hypnotherapy training programs by an agency of the United States Government.

U.S. DEPARTMENT OF EDUCATION
OFFICE OF EDUCATIONAL RESEARCH AND IMPROVEMENT

NATIONAL CENTER FOR EDUCATION STATISTICS

April 27, 1989

Mr. Gil Boyne
Executive Director
American Council of Hypnotist
  Examiners
312 Riverdale Drive
Glendale, California 91204

Dear Mr. Boyne:

Thank you for your presentation at the Review Meeting for the 1990 update of
the Classification of Instructional Programs (CIP) held in Washington, D.C. on
April 5th. Your presentation on Hypnotherapy was both interesting and
informative.

CIP, which is the federally accepted standard used nationally to collect,
report, and interpret data on programs being offered at institutions across the
nation, is periodically reviewed and updated every five years. Program
descriptions are revised to reflect current terminology, new and emerging
programs are added, and programs no longer being offered are deleted.

Based on your presentation and supporting documents, Hypnotherapy will be one
of three new and emerging programs added to CIP under the Health Sciences
category. The program description you submitted has been accepted without
change, justifiable by your role as Executive Director of the primary
organization for the Hypnotherapy profession.

In addition, the names of institutions offering Hypnotherapy, that you provided
to us, will be listed in the Directory of Postsecondary Institutions published
by the National Center for Education Statistics; and the institutions will
become part of the Center's survey universe on postsecondarty education.
Information on location, institutional characteristics, enrollments, program
completions, and tuition and fees, will be collected from each institution.
The statistics will be included in our annual reports and publications.

For your time and effort, The American Council of Hypnotist Examiners will be
acknowledged in the CIP - 1990 publication for its significant contribution.

Sincerely,

Judi Carpenter
CIP Project Director

WASHINGTON, D.C. 20208—

TRANSFORMING THERAPY: A NEW APPROACH TO HYPNOTHERAPY

How the Need Was Created

Modern hypnotherapy has become the most dramatically effective short-term therapy developed to date. The increasing numbers of highly specialized hypnotherapists graduating from state-licensed hypnotherapy schools threaten to undermine the basic assumptions that support traditional psychoanalytic psychotherapy.

These are:

Assumption #1

Everyone needs and can benefit greatly from psychotherapy.

Truth

Almost all of the world's population have not only survived without psychotherapy but most have lived satisfying and productive lives.

Assumption #2

The motivations for human behavior are so complex and deep-rooted that the effectiveness of psychotherapy is directly equated with the extended duration of treatment.

Truth

Therapy is most effective as short-term intervention to produce behavioral change. Therapy of more than limited duration is usually counterproductive because:

    A. It creates psychic dependence on the therapist.

    B. It delays and avoids coping with real-life problems.

    C. It often leads to financial exploitation.

Assumption #3

The theory of the "unconscious" attempts to persuade us that the mythical "id" is a vast repository of destructive, primal energy and that we must spend our lives attempting to tame and re-socialize the "id" or we will live in constant turmoil and upheaval.

Truth

Nowhere in this philosophy is there any hint of the spiritual nature of transformation, or that in each of us is a Divine Intelligence that knows all the answers and is the true essence of our being.

By attaching an atheistic (humanist) superstructure to an unproven, unworkable collection of concepts and labeling the entire structure as "scientific theory," psychoanalysts attempt to retain control of the high ground that once belonged to the holy men.

Secular humanism in psychotherapy has now taken on all the aspects of a religion, but it has no greater preemptive claim to serve as the basis of "healing the soul" than the tenets of the great historic monotheistic religions.

Since morality is the basis of law, whose morality shall we now consult? If someone's values are to prevail, why not ours instead of those of Karl Marx or Sigmund Freud and others who would deny our Divine connection?

The principles upon which America was founded are rooted in a belief in a Supreme Creator ("In God We Trust") and the Divine Nature of man. Now these precious beliefs have been weakened by our acceptance of the new religion of psychoanalytic psychotherapy. When we surrender our belief in God we become free to believe in anyone.

The true ministry of the hypnotherapist is to heal the self-induced blindness that has created a cloud of unknowing.

This realm of the Spirit can best be entered into by hypnotherapists who recognize their work as the "redirecting of an invisible, indefinable spiritual energy to assist another to enter into a State of Grace." We come into a State of Grace through faith in a Higher Power. This faith is acquired through persistent pursuit and continuous reinforcement of a belief until it becomes fixed in the subconscious mind and cannot be changed by intellectual debate or skeptical inquiry. It is a commitment to the "substance of things unseen but perceived through inner spiritual sensing."

HYPNOTHERAPY VS. PSYCHOTHERAPY: IS THERE A REAL DIFFERENCE?

The following ideas are the beginning of a process which will lead to the full identification and recognition of the differences between psychotherapy and hypnotherapy. I urge all practitioners to help me articulate the conceptual, pragmatic and systemic differences. Your contributions are welcomed and recognition will be given as this growing body of material is published.

Phenomena of Trance

1. The development and expression of deductive processing of thought and imagery.

2. The ability to stimulate memory recall and simultaneously revive attached feeling content.

3. An enhanced capacity to quickly develop an emotionalized relationship (rapport) with the helping person.

4. A tremendously heightened capacity to internalize new and different ideas (programming) presented by the helper, utilizing a variety of methods such as implication, supposition, and the use of multiple-level communication (puns, jokes, stories, analogies, and imagery, as well as direct suggestion).

5. Heightened potential for stimulation and manipulation of subconscious memories, scripts, belief systems, and emotionalized attitudes which form the basis for the client's counterproductive behavior.

6. Accessibility to levels of irrational, deductive processing, which generate inhibition and feelings of helplessness expressed in specific forms of maladaptive behavior.

Major Differences Between Psychotherapy and Hypnotherapy

Psychotherapy

Training in psychotherapy begins with and is strongly influenced by Freudian psychoanalytic theories.

Hypnotherapy

Hypnotherapy training begins with the teaching of trance development, followed by the creative utilization of the "phenomena of trance" and a wide variety of uncovering methods for rapid movement toward actualizing goals.

Psychotherapy

Traditional psychotherapy holds a view that virtually everyone has some form of neurosis which emerges as part of a developmental struggle to socialize a primitive, aggressive, and often destructive pool of energy referred to in psychotherapy as the "id" (a theoretic construct).

Hypnotherapy

Hypnotherapy is a naturalistic approach that uses the client's present resources and strengths to further and accomplish meaningful goals.

Psychotherapy

Psychotherapy strongly implies that therapeutic change is usually difficult and time consuming and therefore requires extended therapy (two or more years of regular therapy sessions is not unusual).

Hypnotherapy

Hypnotherapy is usually presented as a dramatically rapid intervention system which strengthens and reshapes the client's feelings of competence and capability.

Part Two

Transforming Therapy at Work:

Transcriptions of Actual Live Case Histories, Presented Verbatim

HYPNOTHERAPY TO OVERCOME MENTAL BLOCKS

The Case of Scotty ("The World's Worst Speller")

A class member reports that he responds well to trance but has no response to programming affirmations (improved spelling).

In three weekly sessions with Gil Boyne before a hypnotherapy class, Scotty discovers how his adult life is contaminated by early childhood programming.

Age regression, Gestalt dialogues, bioenergetic analysis, and "Parts" therapy are utilized.

A four-year follow-up shows an altered perception, a greatly strengthened self-image, no concern with spelling, and a personal transformation.

This case history is fully annotated. When significant material emerges it is identified with bold type as in the following examples:

AN ATTRIBUTION BY PARENT
SELF-REINFORCEMENT
SENSITIZING EVENT
ALTERED PERCEPTION

This provides a continuous outline of process and content and provides a road map to the "therapeutic choices" made by the therapist.

THE CASE OF SCOTTY
The World's Worst Speller
Session One

(The Setting: A Classroom)

(BOYNE ADDRESSES THE AUDIENCE)

BOYNE: Tonight we want to help those who are having trouble evaluating their trance state or who are not going as deeply into hypnosis as they would like to. Who's been having difficulty with that process?

(Scotty, a student from the class, comes forward.)

(BOYNE ADDRESSES SCOTTY)

BOYNE: Will you talk about your responses to hypnosis so far?

SCOTTY: So far my responses have been pretty good, but I don't know how deep I go. I guess I don't have a good comparison. Some of the posthypnotic suggestions I have received haven't really manifested.

BOYNE: Suggestions "received" from whom?

SCOTTY: From another hypnotist. We were working on some anger and some spelling problems, but so far my spelling has not improved.

BOYNE: When was the suggestion given? How far back?

SCOTTY: It was two months.

BOYNE: How often has it been repeated?

SCOTTY: About three times, and then I let it go.

(BOYNE ADDRESSES THE AUDIENCE)

BOYNE: When adults who otherwise show signs of good intelligence and education have a spelling problem, we must look upon the problem as a delusion. They have a delusion they can't spell but they can spell. The evidence of that is that they read newspapers and magazines and books all of the time, and their minds photograph the correct spelling of all the words they say they can't spell many thousands of times. The delusive quality is a belief they acquired at an earlier time.

(BOYNE ADDRESSES SCOTTY)

BOYNE: Do you remember how far back this feeling about not being able to spell goes?

SCOTTY: Grade school.

BOYNE: Can you remember at what grade you had difficulty spelling?

SCOTTY: First or second grade.

BOYNE: Usually the second grade is where it starts. In the first grade there's not too much concern with spelling.

SCOTTY: Right. I did well until the second grade.

BOYNE: How many children were in your family?

SCOTTY: Just me.

BOYNE: What was the educational level of your mother and father?

SCOTTY: My mother had a teacher's credential and my father had a high school education at that point.

BOYNE: You say "at that point." That means he got further education later?

SCOTTY: Yes. That's correct.

BOYNE: It sounds as if you're saying there was a strong emphasis in your family on learning and becoming educated.

SCOTTY: Right, there was a lot of pressure on me.

BOYNE: How did you feel then and how did you respond to that pressure to learn?

SCOTTY: I think I resisted. Yes, I'm sure I resisted.

BOYNE: Did it seem to upset either of your parents when you had difficulty with spelling?

SCOTTY: Yes.

(BOYNE ADDRESSES THE AUDIENCE)

BOYNE: Although I didn't plan to do this, let's see how much we can help this man with his spelling problem, his belief that he is a poor speller. We're going to do that by engaging in a hypnotherapy process, so let's start right now.

(BOYNE ADDRESSES SCOTTY)

BOYNE: Are you ready for me to hypnotize you?

SCOTTY: Yes.

BOYNE: All right. Come right over here. Pull your feet together. Stand relaxed. (Boyne pulls Scotty's head forward as he shouts) SLEEP! Loosely, limply relax. Let every muscle and every nerve grow loose and limp and relaxed. That's fine. Arms limp. The more I rock you, the deeper into hypnosis you're going. Ten, nine, eight, you're drifting down. Seven, six, five, going deeper now. Four, three, two, one. Now sleep deeply. Now I'm going to count from five down to one. As I do, your eyelids lock tightly closed. (Boyne has his left hand on the back of Scotty's neck and his right hand on Scotty's forehead and he gently rotates his head.) Five, eyelids pressing down tightly. Four, they're pressing down and sealing shut. Three, sealing as if they were glued. Two, they're locked. The more you try to open them now, the tighter they're locking closed. One, now try to open your eyelids. They're stuck tight. (Scotty attempts to open his eyelids without success.) Now stop trying. Just relax and go deeper in sleep. That's fine. Now you're much deeper into hypnosis than you were just a few moments ago and going deeper with each easy breath that you take. I'm going to raise both of your arms, and as I drop them, you'll feel a wave of relaxation sweep from the top of your head down to the tip of your toes, and you go much deeper into hypnosis. (Boyne raises Scotty's arms and drops them to Scotty's side.) All right. Get ready now, and just sleep deeply. That's fine. (Boyne places Scotty on the floor.) Loosely, limply relaxed. That's good. Every muscle and every nerve turning loose and letting go. That's wonderful. Relax all over. That's good. There's a feeling that you get.

INTENSIFYING THE PREDOMINANT SUBCONSCIOUS FEELING

It's a feeling that has to do with spelling. It's a feeling of anxiety. It's a feeling of tension. As I count from one up to ten, I want you to become aware of that feeling. All right. One, two, three, the feeling begins to emerge. Four, five, six, growing stronger now. Seven, it's a feeling of not knowing, not being able to spell. Eight, growing stronger and stronger, more intense now. Nine, it's rolling across you in a great wave. Number ten. And now I'm going to count from ten down to one, and as I do, we're going back to an earlier time. It's a time that has to do with this same kind of feeling.

AGE REGRESSION

All right. Ten, nine, eight, now you're drifting back. Seven, six, five, you're growing younger now. Four, your arms and legs are shrinking and you're growing smaller. Three, two, one. (Boyne places his hand on Scotty's forehead.) Where you are now, are you indoors or outside? Make a choice quickly.

SCOTTY: Indoors.

BOYNE: Daytime or nighttime?

SCOTTY: Daytime.

BOYNE: Are you alone or is someone with you?

SCOTTY: Someone's with me.

BOYNE: Who is it that's with you?

SCOTTY: My teacher, my classmates.

BOYNE: You're in school, in the schoolroom. How old are you?

SCOTTY: Seven (in a childish voice).

BOYNE: Seven years old. What grade are you in?

SCOTTY: Second grade.

BOYNE: Second grade. I want you to tell me whatever it is you see, hear, feel, or experience. What's going on?

SCOTTY: The teacher is writing on the blackboard.

BOYNE: Watch the teacher now. See the teacher writing on the blackboard. What are you thinking as the teacher is writing?

SCOTTY: I know how to spell that word.

BOYNE: Say it again.

SCOTTY: I know how to spell that word.

BOYNE: Say it again.

SCOTTY: I know how to spell that word.

BOYNE: What's the teacher doing now?

SCOTTY: She's writing it. She's asking.

BOYNE: How do you feel now that she's asking?

SCOTTY: I'm still angry.

SIGNIFICANT STATEMENT

BOYNE: Finish it like this: "I'm angry because..." or "I'm angry about..." or "I'm angry over...."

SCOTTY: I'm angry because my other teacher embarrassed me.

SENSITIZING EVENT

BOYNE: When I count from three down to one, go to the time and place with the other teacher where you're being embarrassed. Three, two, one. Are you indoors or outside?

SCOTTY: Indoors.

BOYNE: Daytime or nighttime?

SCOTTY: Daytime.

BOYNE: Are you alone or is someone with you?

SCOTTY: Someone is with me.

BOYNE: Who is it that's with you?

SCOTTY: My classmates.

BOYNE: All right. What's happening? Give a report.

SCOTTY: My teacher is angry at me because I won't be quiet.

BOYNE: When I tap your forehead, hear the teacher speaking to you. (Boyne taps Scotty's forehead.) What's she saying now?

SCOTTY: She's saying, "Come over in front of the class."

BOYNE: How does that make you feel?

SCOTTY: I'm embarrassed.

BOYNE: When you feel embarrassed, what do you feel in your body? Go into your body and become aware of that feeling of embarrassment.

SCOTTY: I'm angry.

BOYNE: "I'm angry." Can you tell me where you feel the anger in your body?

SCOTTY: In my stomach.

BOYNE: In your stomach. Can you describe the feeling, like "It feels like..." or "It feels as if..."?

SCOTTY: It feels tight.

BOYNE: All right. A little more description. Tight like what? "Feels as if...feels like...."

SCOTTY: It feels tight like my belt is tight.

BOYNE: Okay. Tight like a belt pulled tight around your waist. How old are you?

SCOTTY: Six.

BOYNE: Six years old. What grade are you in?

SCOTTY: First grade.

BOYNE: First grade. Now you won't stop talking, and so the teacher has called you up in front of the room. Now you're in the front of the room. What is she saying there to you?

SCOTTY: She's putting a towel on my head.

BOYNE: A towel on your head. **Why in the world would she do that?** What does she say as she puts the towel on your head?

SCOTTY: "If you won't stop talking, I'll put this towel over your head."

BOYNE: What are the other kids doing as she puts the towel on your head?

SCOTTY: They're laughing.

BOYNE: Well, of course. **They're laughing at the teacher. What a dumb thing to do, to put a towel on your head.**

REEDUCATION

As you hear them laughing, what are you thinking?

SCOTTY: I'm crying. I don't like it.

BOYNE: How do you feel as you hear the laughter?

SCOTTY: I'm angry.

BOYNE: Let your mind grow clear. (As Boyne says this, he puts his hand on Scotty's head.) Let your mind grow clear. I want you to listen. You see, what the teacher is doing is kind of foolish and dumb because that's not a way to deal with a child who talks too much. All the other kids are laughing because it's kind of funny. They're laughing at her inability to deal with the situation more appropriately, and it looks kind of funny to see someone with a towel on their head. It doesn't mean that you're funny or ridiculous. Also they're a little bit tense. The teacher's angry and they're laughing because they're glad it's not them up there with the towel on their head. You can understand that, can't you?

REEDUCATION—REWRITING THE STORED IMPRINT OR SCRIPT

SCOTTY: Yeah.

BOYNE: Fine. Now when I count to three, we'll go back to the second grade where the teacher is writing on the board. (Boyne taps Scotty's forehead lightly as he counts) One, two, three. Now she's writing the word on the board, and you know you can spell that word. What's going on?

SCOTTY: I can spell it if she would ask me.

BOYNE: If this teacher would ask you, you know that you could spell it. Who is she asking?

SCOTTY: She's asking the girls.

BOYNE: Now what's happening?

SCOTTY: She's getting closer to me.

BOYNE: Here she comes down the line, and now?

SCOTTY: I can spell that word.

BOYNE: Is it your turn yet?

SCOTTY: No. She asked me another word.

BOYNE: A different one. What happened?

SCOTTY: I don't know how to spell it.

BOYNE: Now are you standing or sitting?

SCOTTY: I'm sitting.

BOYNE: You're sitting and you're not spelling the word. What's going on in the room?

SCOTTY: They're laughing.

BOYNE: They're laughing just like they did before when you had the towel on your head?

FEAR OF CRITICISM BY PEERS INTENSIFIED

SCOTTY: Yes.

BOYNE: And how do you feel?

SCOTTY: Embarrassed.

BOYNE: Embarrassed. (Boyne places his hand on Scotty's forehead as he says) Let your mind grow clear. Now just relax and let your mind grow clear until I speak to you again.

(BOYNE ADDRESSES THE AUDIENCE)

BOYNE: We can see this fear of criticism developing. In the first grade the children laughed because of the tension of the situation. Laughter is a discharge of tension, just as crying is. Scotty experienced that as personally embarrassing and humiliating. Now he's focused on spelling one word which he knows and another word is given instead. It comes as a surprise, so he doesn't spell it. It's set in his mind, and also there's a feeling of anger that he keeps referring to. When the kids laugh again it's because they're glad it was he who made the mistake and not they. The anger and the fear of critical evaluation he feels, and the way he interprets the laughter to mean that he looks ridiculous, block his mind and block his ability to remember. Let's see if there are any reinforcing ideas or suggestions at this critical point, which is an **"initial sensitizing event."** Let's go on from there.

INDIRECT REEDUCATION—BOYNE ADDRESSES THE CLASS BUT IS REALLY EXPLAINING TO SCOTTY'S SUBCONSCIOUS MIND

(BOYNE ADDRESSES SCOTTY)

BOYNE: (Boyne taps Scotty's forehead and says) Now I'm speaking to you again. When I count to three, we'll go to a place in which there's some person or some situation in which there is some comment being made about your not spelling.

LOOKING FOR REINFORCEMENT OF EMOTIONALLY BASED BELIEF

All right. One, two, three.

SCOTTY: My mother.

BOYNE: All right. You're home now, is that it?

SCOTTY: Yeah.

BOYNE: What's happening?

SCOTTY: She's telling me that I don't spell very good.

BOYNE: She says you don't spell very good. When I tap your forehead, listen to exactly what she says. (Boyne taps Scotty's forehead.) What is she saying to you?

SCOTTY: She said, "You're a bad speller."

AN ATTRIBUTION

BOYNE: "You're a bad speller." Do you love your mother?

SCOTTY: Yes.

BOYNE: Does your mother love you?

SCOTTY: Yes.

BOYNE: Your mother has a good education. She learned well, didn't she?

SCOTTY: Yes.

BOYNE: Say it again.

SCOTTY: She's a good speller.

BOYNE: She's a good speller and she says that you are a bad speller. Now let your mind grow clear for just a moment. (As Boyne says this, he places his hand on Scotty's head.)

(BOYNE ADDRESSES THE AUDIENCE)

BOYNE: Here we see a *secondary reinforcing event*. Mother is a good speller and is the authority figure in the area of spelling. The authority on spelling says, "You're a bad speller." That's called an "attribution." The mother attributes to this child a functional capacity for misspelling. The question is: How is it integrated? How is it assimilated? How does it become an introject? Let's find out.

INDIRECT REEDUCATION

(BOYNE ADDRESSES SCOTTY)

BOYNE: All right. Mother says you're a bad speller. When I count to three, go ahead to another time where you're having difficulty with spelling. One, two, three. (Boyne taps Scotty's forehead as he counts.) You are having trouble now, the same feelings about spelling. Are you indoors or outside?

SCOTTY: Indoors.

BOYNE: Daytime or nighttime?

SCOTTY: Daytime.

BOYNE: Are you alone or is someone with you?

SCOTTY: Someone's with me.

BOYNE: Who is it that's with you?

SCOTTY: I'm in school with my classmates.

BOYNE: You're in school. How old are you?

SCOTTY: Ten.

BOYNE: Ten years old. What's going on?

SCOTTY: We're practicing spelling.

BOYNE: Do you spell well?

SCOTTY: No.

THE ATTRIBUTION HAS BECOME A FIXED IDEA

BOYNE: You're not a good speller?

SCOTTY: No.

BOYNE: How long have you been having trouble with your spelling?

SCOTTY: Since I've been in school.

SELF-REINFORCEMENT

BOYNE: Now you're practicing spelling. How do you feel?

SCOTTY: I'm just memorizing. I can't remember when I do it that way.

BOYNE: What does that mean?

SCOTTY: Well, if I write it five times, I can remember for a little bit, but then it goes away.

SUBCONSCIOUS ATTITUDE OVERCOMES "ROTE LEARNING"

BOYNE: What does the teacher say about your spelling?

SCOTTY: She grades my papers.

BOYNE: What kind of marks does she give you?

SCOTTY: C.

BOYNE: When I tap your forehead, we'll go back home to mother now. You're ten years old. One, two, three. (Boyne taps Scotty's forehead as he counts.) Now you're with your mother. How does mother feel about your marks on these papers and these marks on your report card?

SCOTTY: She laughs at me.

REINFORCES FEELINGS OF RIDICULE AND EMBARRASSMENT

BOYNE: She laughs at you. Listen again now. Hear her laughing and what she's saying.

SCOTTY: She says I'm a poor speller and she laughs.

BOYNE: What do you think when she laughs at you?

SCOTTY: I don't like it.

BOYNE: What kind of feeling do you feel?

SCOTTY: I get angry.

A DEVELOPED PATTERN OF RESPONSE— ANGER COVERS HURT

BOYNE: Has mother ever made an effort to help you with your spelling?

SCOTTY: Yes.

BOYNE: All right. When I tap your forehead, go to a time when she's attempting to help you with spelling. (Boyne taps Scotty's forehead.) Now you're with your mother. She wants to help you. What's going on?

SCOTTY: She tells me about the rules.

BOYNE: The rules for...?

SCOTTY: Spelling. She says if I know the rules, I can spell.

BOYNE: Do you know the rules?

SCOTTY: Some of them.

BOYNE: Can you spell?

SCOTTY: They don't help.

BOYNE: The rules don't help you to spell?

SCOTTY: No.

NEGATIVE BELIEF, "I CAN'T SPELL," OVERCOMES "RULES"

BOYNE: And mother says if you know the rules, you'll spell, but your discovery is that it's not so. **Mother's not telling you the true facts.**

REEDUCATION—WEAKENING THE ATTRIBUTION

You can learn some of the rules and yet they don't seem to help. Is that true?

SCOTTY: That's true.

BOYNE: Why do you think that is?

SCOTTY: I have trouble remembering all the rules.

BOYNE: Let your mind grow clear. (Boyne places his hand on Scotty's head as he says this.)

(BOYNE ADDRESSES THE AUDIENCE)

BOYNE: **Again we see more reinforcing constantly going on. Mother laughs at him. He feels angry and so when mother attempts to help, and says, "Learn these rules now. You can do that. You can spell. Spell this word," he freezes. His feelings block his ability to recall and he acts out the attribution. He acts out the existing behavior—"I can't spell." Therefore, the expectation is not to spell and that is the self-fulfilling prophecy. Mother behaves in the expected way, she laughs, and he feels embarrassed and angry and guilty, and so the cycle continues. This is the vicious cycle of reinforcement, and worst of all, we now have self-reinforcement. Whenever the subject of spelling comes up, he says, "I've always been a bad speller and I have great trouble remembering."**

INDIRECT REEDUCATION OF THE SUBCONSCIOUS MIND

(BOYNE ADDRESSES SCOTTY)

BOYNE: When I count from one up to four, I want you to go to a time when you're growing older, but still having the problem and the same thoughts and feelings about spelling. One, two, three, four. (Boyne taps Scotty's forehead.) All right. Where you are, are you indoors or outside?

SCOTTY: Indoors.

BOYNE: Is it daytime or nighttime?

SCOTTY: Daytime.

BOYNE: Are you alone or is someone with you?

SCOTTY: Someone is with me.

BOYNE: Who is it that's with you?

SCOTTY: It's my boss.

BOYNE: It's your boss. How old are you?

SCOTTY: I'm forty.

BOYNE: Forty years old. What's going on?

SCOTTY: He's telling me about my spelling.

ADULT REINFORCEMENT

BOYNE: What is he saying?

SCOTTY: He's saying, "Don't write your reports. You can't spell."

SECONDARY PAYOFF

BOYNE: "Don't write any reports because you can't spell." How do you feel about that? What are you thinking as he says that?

SCOTTY: I want to spell.

BOYNE: What else? What are you feeling?

SCOTTY: I feel embarrassed.

BOYNE: Any other feeling?

SCOTTY: Some anger.

BOYNE: All right. Let your mind grow clear. (As Boyne says this, he places his hand on Scotty's head.)

(BOYNE ADDRESSES THE AUDIENCE)

BOYNE: Now the pattern is evident. First the "initial sensitizing event," then many, many reinforcing events.

An authority figure impressing a suggestion which becomes a fixed idea—"You're a poor speller." The mother attributing poor spelling. The self-reinforcement—"I've always had trouble with spelling." Now he's an adult, and at forty he's still getting disapproval from an authority figure, his boss, and because he doesn't understand it, he feels frustrated, angry, and guilty. So how do we deal with that? Well, let's penetrate the veil of unreality. I'll do that again by making contact and talking.

INDIRECT REEDUCATION

(BOYNE ADDRESSES SCOTTY)

BOYNE: (Boyne places his hand on Scotty's head.) All right. I'm speaking to you again now, and I want you to listen carefully. You see, you accepted a belief at a time when your ability to examine suggestions critically was not yet fully developed. And so when mother said, "You can't spell," you accepted that as a true statement. You internalized it. It became a part of your belief system. Then in order to keep that as a fixed belief, you had to constantly act in accordance with that belief because the belief generated a certain energy when a situation of spelling or thoughts about spelling came up, and that energy shaped the way you behaved in a spelling situation. Now something new has happened. You have come to recognize that it's only been an illusion. Because you can spell and you can spell easily. You read the newspapers. You read magazines and you read books, and every time you do, your mind photographs the correct spelling of all the words that you falsely believe you cannot spell.

PROGRAMMING & REEDUCATION

You're going to discover a great veil has been lifted from in front of your eyes. You're going to see clearly some things you saw darkly until just a moment ago. I'm going to count from one up to ten, so you can come up to this place, 1977. One, two, three, four, five, six, seven, eight, nine, ten. This is 1977. It's the month of November. You're a mature, adult personality now, and when I count from three down to one, I want you to look back at the experiences of the boy.

USE YOUR REASONING MIND— RETROFLECTION

See how those early experiences affected him from the first grade forward. See how his mother's suggestions affected him. See what kind of feelings they generated; what kind of thoughts emerged, and what kinds of ideas became fixed. See how that affected his behavior in related areas, and how it affected him as he grew; and how it's even been affecting you today. When you have analyzed that and when the understanding has come from it, raise your hand like this (Boyne demonstrates by lifting Scotty's left hand up.) and we'll talk further about it. Three, two, one. Look back now (Boyne taps Scotty's forehead as he counts.). Look back now and analyze those experiences of the boy.

SCOTTY: (Scotty begins to lift his hand.)

BOYNE: (Boyne takes Scotty's hand and holds it in his own.) All right. Fine. Tell me about it.

SCOTTY: As I looked back, I saw all those incidents. And I began to think I was the world's worst speller. I've said many times, "I'm the world's worst speller."

BOYNE: I want you to say that whole sentence again.

SCOTTY: I've said it many times.

BOYNE: Once again.

SCOTTY: I've said it many times.

BOYNE: Thousands of times, haven't you?

SCOTTY: Thousands of times.

BOYNE: Thousands of times you've reinforced the existing fixed belief that you couldn't spell.

SELF-REINFORCEMENT

SCOTTY: Yes.

BOYNE: Go on.

SCOTTY: And because I was embarrassed, I made a joke of it. And **I got attention,**

SECONDARY PAYOFF

but I don't want that kind of attention now.

BOYNE: Who wants attention for being dumb or behaving in a dumb way or acting dumb?

SCOTTY: I don't want that kind of attention.

BOYNE: That's right. Now what happened to the boy as he grew in terms of his belief and his behaviors?

SCOTTY: I believed what was said—that I was a poor speller.

INTEGRATION

BOYNE: How did it crystallize into a pattern for you as an adult?

SCOTTY: I stayed away from spelling as much as I could.

RECOGNIZES BEHAVIOR PATTERN OF AVOIDANCE

BOYNE: "I avoided spelling whenever I could."

SCOTTY: Yes.

BOYNE: You can understand how the boy acquired those beliefs and those ideas now, can't you?

SCOTTY: Yes.

BOYNE: You can understand the influence of the mother and how the energy coming from her affected him?

SCOTTY: Yes.

BOYNE: How old are you now?

SCOTTY: I'm forty-three.

BOYNE: Forty-three. Is there any need for you to continue functioning as if you were six or eight or ten or any age other than forty-three in relation to spelling?

REQUEST FOR CHANGE

SCOTTY: No.

BOYNE: What then are you ready to do now that's different from the way you function on the basis of those early ideas?

REQUEST FOR CHANGE

SCOTTY: I want to spell.

BOYNE: Haven't you always *wanted* to spell even though you continued not to spell?

SCOTTY: Yes.

BOYNE: What do you want to do now? What kind of behavior do you want to express that's *different* from what you've been doing?

SCOTTY: I *would like* to spell easily and freely.

BOYNE: Didn't you feel you would like to do that earlier?

SCOTTY: Yes.

BOYNE: Then, you're not saying anything different. What do you want to do now that's *different* from the way you thought and felt and acted in the past?

SCOTTY: I've tried many ways. They'd work for awhile and then not work anymore.

BOYNE: There are no ways to spell. You don't try to spell. Either you spell or you don't spell. Which do you want to do?

SCOTTY: I want to spell.

BOYNE: Then what are you going to do about it?

SCOTTY: Spell.

BOYNE: Ah-ha! Say it again.

SCOTTY: Spell.

BOYNE: That's a single word. Link yourself to the word.

SCOTTY: I'm spelling.

BOYNE: Say, "I can spell."

SCOTTY: I can spell.

FREEDOM FROM THE ATTRIBUTION— "YOU CAN'T SPELL."

BOYNE: "I can spell any word that I can see and read."

SCOTTY: I can spell any word that I can see and read.

BOYNE: "And I do it easily."

SCOTTY: And I can do it easily.

PROGRAMMING

BOYNE: Now this time when I have you open your eyes, you're going to feel as if a veil has been lifted, and truly it has. A delusion has been penetrated and punctured. You understand it fully, and with each day you're going to become more aware that the idea you accepted, that you were a bad speller, was simply a lie. It was natural and appropriate for you to accept that programming idea at that early time.

INTEGRATION

It's no longer natural and no longer appropriate. You're a man of great capability, knowledge, education, and training, and you no longer need to sabotage yourself and inhibit yourself or be less than you are by acting out that old childhood pattern. You agree to that, don't you?

SCOTTY: Yes.

BOYNE: All right. When I count from one to five, I want you to let your eyelids open. You're calm, rested, refreshed, relaxed, you feel wonderfully good. Over and over again now, this new clarity of perception about your ability to spell will constantly return to your mind. You'll especially be on guard, so that if ever you feel yourself in an unguarded moment about to express, "I've always been a bad speller," you'll know that's the old childhood lie manifesting itself again. You'll soon cleanse yourself of it easily and quickly. All right. One, slowly, calmly, easily, and gently returning to your full awareness once again. Two, each muscle and nerve in your body is loose and limp and relaxed, and you feel wonderfully good. (Scotty's arm goes down to his side.) Three, from head to toe you're feeling wonderfully perfect in every way. On number four, your eyes begin to feel sparkling clear. On the next number now, let your eyelids open. You're calm, rested, refreshed, relaxed. You feel wonderfully good in every way. Number five, eyelids open now. (Boyne taps Scotty's head.) Take a deep breath. Fill up your lungs and stretch. When you're ready, we'll stand up and talk about that. What do you think of all that went on?

SCOTTY: It was good. I like that.

BOYNE: What did you get from it?

SCOTTY: Well, I really did see the illusion and how it built and how I reinforced it and how I believed it.

BOYNE: How about right now?

SCOTTY: I want to spell. I am a speller.

STATEMENT OF ALTERED PERCEPTION

BOYNE: "Right now" means can you dispel the illusion from your mind in this moment?

SCOTTY: Yeah. (He nods in agreement.)

BOYNE: Thank you. We'll work again next week.

END OF SESSION ONE.

THE CASE OF SCOTTY
The World's Worst Speller
Session Two

(The Setting: A Classroom)

(BOYNE ADDRESSES THE AUDIENCE)

BOYNE: It's one week later and we want to check with our good speller, so we'll invite him to come up.

(BOYNE ADDRESSES SCOTTY)

Welcome. Give a report about your thoughts, feelings, and behavior in the area of spelling or related areas since you were here last Monday.

SCOTTY: After I left here last week, I was spelling everything I heard on the radio. I was spelling it in my head.

ALTERED PERCEPTION

I was spelling things I saw on signs the next day. I felt very confident about my spelling, and it was good. The day after that there was a change and a kind of recurrence of old ideas.

BEGINNING OF REGRESSION TO OLD PATTERNS

BOYNE: Let's stop for a moment.

(BOYNE ADDRESSES THE AUDIENCE)

BOYNE: Sometimes a client may say, "I thought it was working and then it didn't work." But that's not the issue. Either the method works or it doesn't work. If it worked for a day, and he reports that it did, that means that as we deal with it further we can have it work on a permanent basis. If a person despairs in this situation, because the symptom had disappeared for a period of time and now it returns, they may say, "Oh, that didn't work." That's not true. How can the person forget the period, however brief, of altered function? There's no way he can erase from his memory the fact that for twenty-four hours he could spell anything that he heard.

(BOYNE ADDRESSES SCOTTY)

BOYNE: Please continue.

SCOTTY: I thought it over, and it seemed to me that the key to proper spelling is the idea that you gave me that the words are photographed in my memory, and it's a matter of putting them out and getting myself out of the way so that they come out. I was thinking of making a tape to reinforce that and listen to it once or twice a day. But it's like the old ways are pulling me back.

RESISTANCE TO CHANGE

BOYNE: That's a good description. He says, "Like the old ways, the old ideas." Actually it is the habituated response: "I behave in this way in this situation because I behave in this way in this situation." That's the only reason and that creates a pull. William James said: "All human beings resist change because we cling to familiar patterns and in the familiar we find our security." When we make an adaptation, as you did, you learned to avoid spelling. We make an adaptation and if the adaptation enables us to function without too much suffering, then we cling to the adaptation.

Why go through the process of tearing ourselves from security to an insecure position when there's not that much suffering? But the answer is that we cannot grow, expand, and realize as long as we have an inhibitory voice which says, "I'm not so smart because I can't spell." Then we're not all that we can be. The goal is to recognize what kind of a price you pay to cling to the old security of that familiar and habitual response which is, "I can't spell, I'm not a good speller." Let's talk about that. What is the price you pay if you stay unchanged?

SCOTTY: The price I pay is embarrassment whenever I get into a situation where my spelling is checked out.

BOYNE: Not just embarrassment, it's the worst kind of embarrassment because it's the embarrassment of catastrophic expectations. That means, every time a situation occurs in which you may be called upon to spell, in fantasy you see the worst happening, and indeed it does happen. What does the boss tell you?

SCOTTY: Don't write any reports.

BOYNE: "Don't write any reports because you're such a terrible speller." And that's pretty embarrassing.

SCOTTY: (He nods in agreement.)

BOYNE: Now these reports you were told not to write, how will they be written instead if you don't write them?

SCOTTY: Somebody else will do it.

AVOIDANCE OF RESPONSIBILITY

BOYNE: All right. So that's a possibility. Then where are some other places in which you might experience that embarrassment? Do you have children?

SCOTTY: Yes.

BOYNE: Is it a family script to say, "Dad is a terrible speller"?

SCOTTY: It's the one that I reinforce. The children are good spellers.

BOYNE: But they don't come to you if they're not sure of how to spell a word?

SCOTTY: That's right.

BOYNE: They go to their mother.

SCOTTY: Yeah, for sure!

(BOYNE ADDRESSES THE AUDIENCE)

BOYNE: Now that's interesting because with my daughter, I let her know that I had been a spelling champion in school and that I was very bright and she was very bright. In the fifth grade, they were giving an award at school for creative writing, a $5 cash prize for the best story, and my daughter won it. Maybe she knew she was getting the award that day, but she called home to say she had forgotten something and would I please bring it to her. Just as I got there, she said, "Oh, Dad, I just won the $5 award," and everyone was very excited. Then she said, "But of course, I take after my dad and he was the champion speller." You see? Now the reason I was very deliberate about doing that is because my wife says, "I've always been a terrible speller." She's a well educated person and has a college degree. Yet, she claims she's a terrible speller and says, "I misspell a lot of words." So rather than take the risk of having my daughter identifying with her, quite early I established that she was like me in the area of spelling. And that's the way it's working out—she's a terrific speller.

(BOYNE ADDRESSES SCOTTY)

BOYNE: The first day passed; that was Saturday. On Sunday you began to feel some of the old pulls, and then came Monday and Tuesday, tell us about those days.

SCOTTY: Well, I had been writing some information on positive suggestions and I found that to get through that material, I chose to set aside everything else just so I could finish these positive suggestions.

BOYNE: You gave the development and writing of the programming and affirmations a high priority over everything else.

SCOTTY: Yes I did.

BOYNE: You didn't avoid taking some corrective steps, but rather gave it a high priority and got to it and stayed with it. How did the process go once you got into it? Was it difficult, easy, or somewhere in between?

SCOTTY: The writing was easy as usual.

BOYNE: How about the spelling?

SCOTTY: That's what I did, I stayed away from it. I just wrote it the way it came out, and I'd check it later. I really did put the whole issue of spelling aside.

BOYNE: "I didn't sit in judgment on whether or not I was spelling correctly."

SCOTTY: That's right.

BOYNE: "I dealt with content and not with spelling."

SCOTTY: That's right.

BOYNE: That's a positive step. What else?

SCOTTY: I know the way that I can regain what happened right after this session and the next day was to reinforce that idea of the photographic memory—it's right there. I was talking with somebody at the break and they had the same difficulty with spelling but found this way by themselves. It had never occurred to me. I think that's the way to do it.

(BOYNE ADDRESSES THE AUDIENCE)

REEDUCATION AND INDIRECT PROGRAMMING

BOYNE: **The process is under way and you can hear it in Scotty's report. There's no way he can ever go back unless the secondary gains were really strong enough. There are a number of reasons (gains) for clinging to a psychic pattern, such as maintaining a pattern to get attention or sympathy, to punish oneself or to punish others, to avoid responsibility of one kind or another, or to act out an identification with someone. The secondary gain quite often can be coincidental. For example, by not doing** my homework, I gain some free time to go out to play; but I have to pay the price when I go to school on Monday because the teacher is going to say, "Where is your homework?" A sign of maturity is the measurement of the price that we pay for what we get.

SCOTTY: (He nods in agreement.)

BOYNE: We decide if we're willing to pay the price and if it is worth it. Then if we say, "Yes, it's worth it. Yes, I want it. Yes, I can pay the price and, yes, I'm willing to pay it," we can act upon it, and then we have let the adult make the decision rather than having the adapted child or the critical parent force us to make a decision.

SCOTTY: (He nods in agreement.)

BOYNE: Now we'll do a little more work here, more of what we did before, and this time, rather than twenty-four hours of that feeling of euphoria and freedom from that cloud of unreality that says, "I can't spell," we're going to dispel the cloud a little farther, and if there is some kind of emotional rejection, the cloud will be much thinner this time with more and more holes in it.

(BOYNE ADDRESSES SCOTTY)

BOYNE: Is that agreeable to you?

SCOTTY: Uh-huh.

BOYNE: Just put your hands on your lap. Look at me now. Take a deep breath. Exhale slowly. SLEEP NOW! (Boyne snaps his fingers and pulls Scotty forward slightly. Boyne has his right hand on Scotty's forehead, rocking it as he says) Let your eyelids close down. Let every muscle and nerve grow loose, limp, and relaxed and feel good all over now. The more I rock you, the deeper into hypnosis you're going. I'm going to raise your hand. I'll raise it by taking hold of your thumb. It will hang limply in my fingers. When I drop your hand, it drops limply like a wet, limp dish rag, and you'll feel a wave of relaxation sweep from the top of your head down to the tip of your toes.

All right. Now the other hand, and we get another wave of relaxation and you go much deeper. (Boyne does the same thing with Scotty's left hand—he picks it up by the thumb and then drops it into Scotty's lap.) Once again, I'm going to count from one up to ten and as I do, you're going to get back in touch with the feeling that is very familiar to you.

It's a feeling of embarrassment, a feeling of mortification, a feeling of fear and anxiety. It has to do with feeling that you will not, I repeat, that you will not be able to spell in a given situation.

INTENSIFICATION OF THE UNDERLYING FEELING

All right. One, two, three. Now the feeling begins emerging. Four, you see yourself trying to spell and not doing it and they're laughing at you. Five, six, you hear your mother's laughter as she says you can't spell. Six, she says you're a terrible speller. Seven, you hear the children in school laughing at you. Eight, you avoid spelling because you don't want to feel that mortification and anxiety. Nine, the wave grows stronger and stronger. Now it's like the floodgates on a dam opening up as a great wave of feeling floods across you. Number ten.

AGE REGRESSION

Now I'm going to count from ten down to one. As I do we'll go back to an earlier time. It's a time that has to do with this same kind of feeling. All right. Ten, nine, eight, now you're drifting back. Seven, six, five, you're growing younger now. Four, your arms and legs are shrinking and you're growing smaller. Three, two, one. (Boyne taps Scotty's forehead.) All right. Where you are, are you indoors or outside? Make a choice, quickly.

SCOTTY: I'm outside.

BOYNE: Daytime or nighttime?

SCOTTY: Daytime.

BOYNE: Are you alone or is someone with you?

SCOTTY: By myself.

BOYNE: How old are you?

SCOTTY: Seven.

BOYNE: Seven years old. How do you feel?

SCOTTY: I don't want to go to school. I don't, I don't.

BOYNE: You're seven years old, and you don't want to go to school. What is it that you're thinking about?

SCOTTY: I don't, I don't want to go to class.

BOYNE: Do you feel that way every day or is there something in school today that makes you feel that way?

SCOTTY: I'm going to have a test today.

BOYNE: What will the test be in today?

SCOTTY: Spelling.

BOYNE: Are you a good speller?

SCOTTY: No.

BOYNE: When did you learn that you were not a good speller? When I tap your forehead, go to that time when you made the discovery that you're not a good speller. (Boyne taps Scotty's forehead.) Where are you now?

SCOTTY: I'm in the second grade.

BOYNE: Second grade. What's going on?

SCOTTY: The teacher's teaching spelling.

BOYNE: How is she teaching? What is the method? Does she spell the word aloud? Does she write it on the board? Does she have you read it from the book? What is she doing?

SCOTTY: We have a book.

BOYNE: A book. Now look at the book and open the book to where she's telling you to read. What is the word that you see there?

SCOTTY: Butler.

BOYNE: What's the teacher doing now? What's happening?

SCOTTY: She writes it on the board.

BOYNE: Can you see it on the board?

SCOTTY: Yeah.

BOYNE: And now?

SCOTTY: I know how to spell that.

BOYNE: Can you spell it for me now?

SCOTTY: Capital B-U-T-L-E-R.

BOYNE: That's right! You're a good speller. Now what's happening?

SCOTTY: There's other words.

BOYNE: Are they on the board as well?

SCOTTY: They're in the book.

BOYNE: In the book. All right.

SCOTTY: They're easy.

BOYNE: Easy word. Pick out an easy word and spell it for me, please.

SCOTTY: Cat. C-A-T.

BOYNE: C-A-T. That's right. That is a very good word, and

you spelled it very well. What's the teacher doing now?

SCOTTY: She's—she wants me to spell some other words. I didn't study. I don't know those.

BOYNE: I see. How do you feel as she asks you to spell a word you haven't studied?

SCOTTY: I'm scared.

BOYNE: Did the teacher assign that word for study? How did it happen that she's asking you to spell a word that you didn't study?

SCOTTY: Well, she assigned it.

BOYNE: I see, but somehow you didn't get to study it; is that right?

SCOTTY: I didn't study.

BOYNE: Well, if you don't study a word, you can't be expected to spell it. Now what's happening? She has asked you to spell this word. What's happening?

SCOTTY: I don't know how to spell it.

BOYNE: All right. Do you make an effort to spell it?

SCOTTY: Yes.

BOYNE: Make the effort now. Let me hear you.

SCOTTY: A-P-P-E-L-A-C-I.

BOYNE: What does that spell?

SCOTTY: I don't know. I don't know how to spell it.

BOYNE: All right. And what do you hear? What does the teacher say? What do the other kids do?

SCOTTY: She said I didn't capitalize.

BOYNE: You didn't capitalize. How do you feel?

SCOTTY: I'm angry.

BOYNE: Angry. When I count to three, I'm going to give you an opportunity to do something that you need to do. You'll be seated in a chair and about six feet out in front of you is the teacher. Now you'll be all alone. It's after school, and you can talk to her. All right. One, two, three. Now there's the teacher. I want you to talk to her and tell her how you feel. How do you call her? Do you call her "teacher" or by her name?

SCOTTY: I call her teacher.

BOYNE: Talk to her: "Teacher, I want to tell you how I feel." Tell her now.

GESTALT DIALOGUE

SCOTTY: I don't like her.

BOYNE: Tell her that.

SCOTTY: I don't like you.

BOYNE: All right. Be the teacher. Your student says he doesn't like you. Answer him.

SCOTTY: (As the teacher) He doesn't have to like me. He just has to do the work.

BOYNE: Say that to him.

SCOTTY: (As the teacher—sternly) You don't have to like me, just do the work.

BOYNE: All right. Be the boy. Teacher says you don't have to like her, but you have to do the work.

SCOTTY: Well, I don't like you (sullenly).

BOYNE: Say it again.

SCOTTY: I don't like you (louder).

BOYNE: Again.

SCOTTY: I don't like you (louder).

BOYNE: Tell her what it is that she does or doesn't do that makes you feel that way.

INTENSIFYING THE FEELING

SCOTTY: She's mean.

BOYNE: Say that to her.

SCOTTY: You're mean.

BOYNE: Again.

SCOTTY: You're mean.

BOYNE: Be the teacher. The boy says you're mean. Answer that.

SCOTTY: (As the teacher) I'm not mean to you.

BOYNE: Say it again.

SCOTTY: (As the teacher) I'm not mean to you.

BOYNE: Be the boy.

SCOTTY: Yes you are.

BOYNE: Tell her how she's mean: "You're mean when you..."

SCOTTY: You're mean when you ask me to spell and I don't know the words, and I'm scared of you too.

BOYNE: Be the teacher.

SCOTTY: (As the teacher) Well, I want you to be scared of me. That's the only way you'll work.

BOYNE: Be the boy.

SCOTTY: Well, I don't work when I'm scared.

BOYNE: Say that again.

SCOTTY: I don't work when I'm scared.

BOYNE: Again, louder.

SCOTTY: I won't work when I'm scared!

BOYNE: One more time.

SCOTTY: I won't work when I'm scared. (Forcefully)

BOYNE: Be the teacher.

SCOTTY: (As the teacher—strongly) Well, by God, you're going to work.

BOYNE: Be the boy.

SCOTTY: I won't.

BOYNE: Again.

SCOTTY: I won't.

BOYNE: Again.

SCOTTY: I won't. (As Scotty is saying this his voice is getting louder.)

BOYNE: Again.

SCOTTY: I WON'T!

BOYNE: Let your mind grow clear.

(BOYNE ADDRESSES THE AUDIENCE)

BOYNE: There's the secondary payoff. He expresses his defiance and concealed anger, but he doesn't spell.

(BOYNE ADDRESSES SCOTTY)

BOYNE: I'm going to count from one up to ten. Come up to 1977. One, two, three, four, five, six, seven, eight, nine, ten. This is 1977. Now once again, look back. I'll count from three down to one. Use your adult reasoning mind, analyze the experience of the boy. Analyze what he did; what ideas came to him as a result of doing it; how he felt and how those ideas affected his behavior in the area of spelling and other related areas; how those same ideas affected him as he grew; and how they may be affecting you today. When you're ready to talk about it, just raise your hand like this (Boyne picks up Scotty's right hand to demonstrate) and we'll discuss it. All right. Three, two, one. Now look back and analyze that experience. Good, that took you about ten seconds. So let's go on from there. What do you want to tell me?

SCOTTY: I see that my refusal to spell is a defiance towards authority.

BOYNE: You're an adult now. Who's the authority? Where is the authority?

SCOTTY: I'm the authority.

BOYNE: The authority is in you. So when you defy authority, you defy one of your own ego states. The parent that says, "You should spell." A man your age "should be a better speller." And then you defy that "should" by saying, "Yes, but I can't."

SCOTTY: That's right.

BOYNE: But we know now it's not, "I can't." What is it?

SCOTTY: Won't.

BOYNE: "I won't." Please go on.

SCOTTY: I have refused to spell many times and have used it— to make people angry. I've used it to feel a sense of power. I have felt guilty about it.

BOYNE: When I count to three, you may open your eyes. When you open your eyes, I want you to stand up and look at the group, and I want you to say this to them. "Anytime I decide I won't spell, there's not a thing in all this world that you can do to get me to spell." Really sell it to them so they'll be convinced. All right. One, two, three. Open your eyes. Stand up now and tell them about that.

SCOTTY: When I decide not to spell, there isn't a thing in the world that anybody here can do to change that.

(BOYNE ADDRESSES THE AUDIENCE)

BOYNE: Do you agree with that out there? Tell him.

AUDIENCE: You're in charge.

BOYNE: Again.

AUDIENCE: You're in charge.

(BOYNE ADDRESSES SCOTTY)

BOYNE: All right. Just stand now and SLEEP! (Boyne snaps his fingers and places his hand on Scotty's forehead as he tells him to sleep.) Now this time when you open your eyes, you're going to feel that same feeling you had Saturday of last week—the feeling that you could spell any word because you can; that feeling of euphoria; the feeling that the veil is lifted and the delusion has been penetrated and dispelled. You can stand in front of this group as a champion speller because you want to; and you can spell any word they ask you to spell, not because they ask you to, but because you can show them the choice is yours. You can either spell or not spell, and right now you'll show them that you spell because it's your choice. All right. Open your eyes (Boyne taps Scotty's forehead as he says this) and be a champion speller.

(BOYNE ADDRESSES THE AUDIENCE)

BOYNE: Now you can choose any word and this gentleman will spell it for you right now. Raise your hand if you have a word for him to spell. Yes, sir.

AUDIENCE: Program.

SCOTTY: P-R-O-G-R-A-M.

BOYNE: Yes, sir.

AUDIENCE: Rhythm.

SCOTTY: R-H-Y-T-H-M.

BOYNE: (Boyne points to a woman.)

AUDIENCE: Appalachia

SCOTTY: Capital A-P-P-A-L-A-C-H-I-A.

BOYNE: (Boyne points to another student in the audience.)

AUDIENCE: Therapeutic.

SCOTTY: T-H-E-R-A-P-E-U-T-I-C.

BOYNE: Another word. Compromise.

SCOTTY: C-O-M-P-R-O-M-I-S-E.

BOYNE: Do you have a word for this man?

AUDIENCE: Constantinople.

BOYNE: Constantinople. That's one they always try to trick you on.

SCOTTY: Capital C-O-N-S-T-A-N-T-I-N-O-P-L-E.

BOYNE: All right. Another word out there. Yes, sir.

AUDIENCE: Believe.

SCOTTY: Believe. B-E-L-I-E-V-E.

AUDIENCE: Receive.

SCOTTY: R-E-C-E-I-V-E.

AUDIENCE: Alice.

SCOTTY: Alice. Capital A-L-I-C-E.

BOYNE: That's right. Now give them a message about your spelling.

SCOTTY: It's there any time I want it.

BOYNE: Say, "Any time I want to spell, I'll spell."

SCOTTY: Any time I want to spell, I'll spell.

BOYNE: "And any time I don't want to spell, I won't spell."

SCOTTY: Any time I don't want to spell, I won't spell.

BOYNE: All right. Show your appreciation to this gentleman.

AUDIENCE: (They applaud Scotty.)

(BOYNE ADDRESSES SCOTTY)

BOYNE: (He snaps his fingers and says) Open your eyes now. You're fully aware, fully aware. Well, champ, tell us about your spelling ability. How does that feel?

SCOTTY: It feels good. It feels effortless.

BOYNE: You no longer have to use those old, childish methods, do you?

SCOTTY: No.

BOYNE: Let me give you another message for the group. Stand up. Look at them and say, "If I feel I need to defy you, I'll defy you in an adult way."

SCOTTY: If I feel I need to defy you, I'll defy you in an adult way.

BOYNE: How does that feel?

SCOTTY: That feels good.

BOYNE: Please sit down again. **You can give up that old childhood pattern of saying, "I'll defy you by not spelling," or "I'll show you." You can never show us anything because we can only make decisions about you based on where we are and how we experience you. No matter how close we become, we'll never experience all of you. We'll experience some of the appearance of you; and if you appear to be dumb at times, that may be part of the way we read you or we may become confused about you—He doesn't look dumb but he acts dumb. Shall I take advantage of him or shall I play the role of educator and let him defy me? Shall I play "rescuer" and say, "I'll teach you how to spell— I'll do what others have failed to do"? Then I have to get involved with a wide range of possibilities that are a waste of time. I want to relate to you and I want to give you love, affection, approval. All those other things just obscure the issue.**

REEDUCATION

SCOTTY: Uh-huh.

BOYNE: Thank you very much.

(Boyne and Scotty shake hands.)

SCOTTY: Thank you.

(BOYNE ADDRESSES THE AUDIENCE)

BOYNE: Now the question arises, in the second grade do they give words for spelling such as Appalachia? Unlikely, but you must remember not to get caught up again in the fantasy. The fantasy is that he's back in the second grade, but he's not really. He's vividly remembering being in the second grade. The issue is not "is that really the way it was?" or "is that the way they have come to believe that it was?" The issue is that whatever they report is truth for them and that's what must be dealt with therapeutically. Appalachia could have been a word that this man failed to spell in the fifth grade, but it's locked into a little pigeon hole in the mind called "Words I failed to spell in class when I was called on." That's all that it means. He is not in the second grade; he's in front of this class vividly remembering experiences of the second grade.

In addition, there is a component that enables him to be very close to that experience emotionally and to feel again the quality of the emotion he experienced then. He said, "I feel angry," and I helped him to feel the anger more by having him express it more strongly in the dialogue. What did you get from the dialogue?

AUDIENCE: I thought there was a great deal of interesting content there.

BOYNE: Discuss it more fully!

AUDIENCE: His perception of the teacher from the teacher's point of view, and that the motivating factor is fear.

BOYNE: He is remembering the teacher as a very aggressive, dictatorial, repressive personality who said, "You'll do it because I say so." That didn't sit very well with him at that time. It doesn't sit very well with most children, but based on his psychodynamics, that upset him. He acknowledges now that he got back at that "top dog" attitude by not spelling, which is a different set of ideas than last week's session dealt with. Last week was a lot of scripting, and now we see a new level which was uncovered—this idea of secondary gain.

AUDIENCE: In the catharsis when he expresses this energy, is there going to be any residual energy left? Is he going to get rid of all of those negative feelings that he had back in the second grade or are they going to start building up again when he runs into any kind of authority?

BOYNE: Habituated responses are really established neural pathways, or behavioral responses that are etched in patterns and stored in the neural pathways in the brain. We dig a groove and the energy fires down that groove each time, and each time the nervous system reacts in a given way, it becomes easier for it to react the same way the next time. That's how the patterns of reaction are formed, both good and bad. We can't undo the old neural pathway. We can't erase it; we can't get rid of it. We just establish a new neural pathway. How does a person who has the habituated responses of half a million cigarettes smoked over a forty-year period establish new neural pathways in all those situations where he formerly smoked? He starts, that's how.

When he thinks, "I finished this cup of coffee and I didn't light a cigarette," he's establishing a new neural pathway. Slowly the new neural pathways become established. The new patterns don't have to be repeated as often as the old ones in order to start being a behavioral determinant because you have energy that reminds you. It says, "This is what I want to do until it becomes involuntary." After a person has been relieved of compulsive behavior and delusive beliefs, are they fully dispelled or is there a predisposition for regression? Yes, there is a predisposition for regression because the old neural pathway still exists.

When very intense stress comes upon the organism, the potential for regression exists at that time of heavy stress. Let's say the symptoms are headaches and when certain kinds of stressful situations occur this patient gets a headache. Now through the therapy the headaches have spread out and rather than having them every evening, they've gone to every third evening and then once a week and now they're down to once a month, and they're very faint. Suddenly the client reports to you that they have a terrible headache. It's lasted for three days; it's worse than it ever was; and they say, "I thought it was working but I see now it's worse than ever." That's a regression, and you must tell them, "This will pass and each regression that you have will be at a greater distance from the last one and will be less intense, less severe. You can never go back to where you were because you remember the results that you've had and you cannot erase that memory."

Scotty, we'll work again next week.

END OF SESSION TWO.

THE CASE OF SCOTTY
The World's Worst Speller
Session Three

(The Setting: A Classroom)

(BOYNE ADDRESSES THE AUDIENCE)

BOYNE: This is the third session of our ongoing hypnotherapy of the man who called himself "the world's worst speller."

(BOYNE ADDRESSES SCOTTY)

Would you come up, Scotty. It's been two weeks since we started working on your delusion. Tell me about the past seven days.

SCOTTY: The past seven days I have had sporadic times when my spelling was very good, and other times it's like I've gone back to the old way.

BOYNE: In the seven days sometimes it was very good, sometimes it was not so good, and sometimes it was terrible.

SCOTTY: That's right.

BOYNE: How was that different than it was fifteen days ago?

SCOTTY: The difference is that I now know that I can spell perfectly if I want to.

BOYNE: How do you know that?

SCOTTY: Because I've done it.

BOYNE: Because you do it some of the time.

SCOTTY: That's right.

BOYNE: And fifteen days ago you didn't do it at any time.

SCOTTY: That's right.

BOYNE: It was terrible all of the time, wasn't it?

SCOTTY: Uh-huh. But now I've noticed that there is a **kind of a trigger or something that allows me to spell perfectly.**

SIGNIFICANT STATEMENT

(BOYNE ADDRESSES THE AUDIENCE)

BOYNE: That's something to look for. He said, "There is a trigger that allows me to spell perfectly." If there is a trigger that allows him to spell, then there still is an inhibition that he believes prevents him from doing it. There's a positive trigger and a negative trigger, and that's something we can search for in the therapy.

(BOYNE ADDRESSES SCOTTY)

BOYNE: You say there is a trigger. I'm sure you know more about it. What kind of a feeling is the trigger? "When I get this feeling then I know that I can spell." Describe it please.

SCOTTY: On a feeling level...there's a knowing. When it's not in effect, I'm guessing.

BOYNE: "I'm unsure," or "uncertain."

SCOTTY: That's right.

BOYNE: I'd like to see if we can find some correlation between your function of spelling and your dysfunction of nonspelling. Does stress, nervousness, or nervous tension have to do with it? Can you find a common denominator that has to do with situations in which the insecurity or uncertainty exists, or is there a common denominator when the knowing exists?

SCOTTY: I really hadn't thought about it. Most of the time when I spell, I'm conscious of the fact that I have spelled very poorly.

BOYNE: You mean that now you're more conscious of misspelling than you used to be, or is it the same?

SCOTTY: I'm more conscious of the spelling now because we

have been working with it. But I'm even more upset when I'm in front of a group or having my work checked by my boss, and the intensity is greater.

BOYNE: When there is a potential for criticism, then you feel more anxious.

SCOTTY: Uh-huh.

BOYNE: Now let's stop for just a moment.

(BOYNE ADDRESSES THE AUDIENCE)

BOYNE: That's very interesting. It means that the defenses that he used earlier to protect himself against his fear of criticism and critical evaluation are not operative anymore. In some way we've stripped away those defenses so that now he feels more anxiety about not spelling.

(BOYNE ADDRESSES SCOTTY)

BOYNE: Am I saying it right?

SCOTTY: Sometimes if I just go ahead—as when I gave a lecture and I used the blackboard, and I misspelled two words. I didn't even think about it. I was working, I just went right through it. After it was over, I said, "Did I misspell any words?" I went back and checked and I had. That's why I say it's as if it can be put aside.

BOYNE: Good. That means as you were writing on the board, you weren't thinking, "I hope I spell all those words correctly."

SCOTTY: No, I wasn't.

BOYNE: The anxiety factor is diminished. When you discovered that you had misspelled a couple of words, how did you feel then?

SCOTTY: I was disappointed that I did not spell perfectly, and I covered it up with humor.

BOYNE: How did you do that?

SCOTTY: Well, I—I talked to a couple of the people that were standing around, and I said, "Did I spell all the words correctly?" They said, "No, you misspelled two." I looked up at everyone and I laughed, and I kind of covered my embarrassment with laughter.

BOYNE: Did you make any statement such as, "Well, I'm a terrible speller"?

SCOTTY: No, I didn't say that.

BOYNE: Or, "Only two wrong words is pretty good for a lousy speller like me."

SCOTTY: No, I didn't say that.

BOYNE: Good. Is it likely you would have said that in the past?

SCOTTY: Yes.

BOYNE: Last month?

SCOTTY: Yes, I would have reinforced it.

(BOYNE ADDRESSES THE AUDIENCE)

BOYNE: You see now how the dynamics are changing.

(A QUESTION FROM THE AUDIENCE)

STUDENT: Are you saying, "I'm the world's worst speller," is a defense?

BOYNE: One of his defenses.

SCOTTY: That was the reinforcement in the laughter and any way that I could manage my discomfort.

BOYNE: Yes. The defense part of that statement is, "There's no need for you to be critical of my poor spelling. I acknowledge I'm the world's worst speller. How can you criticize me for something I've already told you?"

(BOYNE ADDRESSES SCOTTY)

BOYNE: Then they said, "You spelled two words incorrectly." How did you feel then?

SCOTTY: I was embarrassed.

BOYNE: You said earlier, "I was embarrassed because I wasn't perfect."

SCOTTY: That's right.

BOYNE: Let's stop for a moment with that.

(BOYNE ADDRESSES THE AUDIENCE)

REEDUCATION

BOYNE: One of the defenses against the intense fear of criticism is perfectionism. "If I do it perfectly, I can't be criticized." But the problem with perfectionism is that the perfectionist never gets any satisfaction. Even when there's a measurable improvement, if there's no satisfaction, no feeling of accomplishment and achievement, then the negative pool of energy that creates the anxiety will remain. The same characteristics remain and the voice which says he wasn't perfect continues to speak. If "I'm the world's worst speller," represented zero on a scale and if the ability to spell all the words that he encountered were one hundred, then we must be sure that he doesn't believe that he will leap from zero to one hundred in a brief period of time, because that's not the way it works. He has already made a major leap because he now spells a lot of words he always knew how to spell but didn't believe that he could spell. Let's say he leaped from zero to forty-five. Now he has to get the feel of being at that plateau for a while with a reduction of anxiety, with altered secondary payoffs and getting those things done in a new way.

He knows that if he needs to defy, he'll defy in an adult pattern. He'll assert himself in other ways. He'll get attention in ways other than through not spelling, and by taking away those payoffs, there will be a little bit of anxiety. It's like, "How do I get that same laughter, that kind of jovial feeling that I used to get when I made a joke of this? How do I get the attention? How do I fix them like I used to fix the teacher who said, 'You'll do it because I said so.'?" He has to find new ways so there's some open ground between where he's been and where he's going.

The process of change is a mystical process. No one understands it, and when you get to the other side, it is just as difficult to go back. The only way he can go back to where he was is if he sells himself back, but he can never go all the way back because he always remembers where he's been. When he gets to the feeling of being at level forty-five, then he may decide that he can go to sixty. When you stay a while at that level, you can go to sixty. Now let's say he never gets to ninety-five. Let's say that, for whatever reason, he gets up to eighty, don't you think he feels a remarkable, extraordinary, incredible change if he started at zero and now he's up to eighty? But if he remains perfectionistic and says, "Oh, I missed a word," and becomes intensely self-critical again, then he sabotages himself and his progress. He attacks it and says, "It's not really worthwhile because if it had been a really successful process of change, I would be perfect."

SCOTTY: (He nods in agreement.)

(BOYNE ADDRESSES SCOTTY)

BOYNE: You're not going to do all those things to yourself, are you?

SCOTTY: No.

BOYNE: All right. Now give a report to us about where you've gone from where you were—a comprehensive report about the growth, movement, and expansion that you have had in two weeks.

SCOTTY: Well, I learned that I had conditioned myself not to spell properly because I was using it as a defense and to get back at authority in a defiant way. I learned under hypnosis that I could spell very well. I also became aware that it isn't magic, that there have to be some changes made in my thinking, because I can feel myself blocking.

BOYNE: That's a good description. You said, "It isn't magic." The whole process is effecting changes in your thinking.

SCOTTY: Uh-huh.

BOYNE: That's what hypnosis is all about. The purpose of hypnosis is to effect changes in the way you think in a given situation. You see, when the impotent male is in a situation where sexual lovemaking might occur, he holds a thought, "I'm going to fail," and that's what happens. It becomes a self-fulfilling prophecy. Now, he can do one of two things. Either he can find ways to avoid sexual situations, such as not feeling good, or staying up late and watching television, or maybe he's creative enough and secure enough that he doesn't get that upset. He might decide that he can still be loving and make loving contact in other ways and not be too concerned. If he does that, it's quite conceivable that it won't become a chronic pattern, that he will begin to have a success here and there which will lead to more success without therapy. But, as long as he holds the expectation to fail, he will fail.

I had a client whose wife had been very ill and in a wheelchair for three years before her death, and during that period they weren't able to experience marital intercourse. Then she died and he felt very guilty. Often when people are chronically ill, those closest to them experience great feelings of rage, helplessness, and then guilt because there's great difficulty in having to take care of a chronically ill person until they die. Whatever the reasons, he was now incapable of having sexual relations with a woman.

He came to me and he said, "This is the problem. I have friends who invite me to social gatherings and dinners and they invite single ladies for me to meet— you know, matchmaking. I won't go anymore because I'm not going to be embarrassed, mortified, and humiliated again in that way. A friend of mine told me about this good-looking woman and he wants me to meet her. He and his wife want to invite us to dinner the day after tomorrow, but I'm not going to go."

I said, "The reason that you're embarrassed and mortified is that you're developing a situation in which you build a certain expectancy. Suppose the situation were changed and you altered the expectancy." He said, "What do you mean?" I said, "Suppose you met this lady and made a date with her, and when you're alone with her an intimate situation develops and you might wind up in the bedroom. At this point you alter your behavior and you say to her, 'Before we go on, I want to tell you I have a problem. I'm working on it clinically with a therapist and very shortly I expect I'll be over it. I'm telling you now because if I fail to respond in a way that you might expect, I want you to know it's not because I don't find you attractive or lovable or exciting. It's my problem.'"

I said, "You see, if you'll do that, then you give the lady an opportunity to process that input, and you won't feel as mortified whatever happens."

He thought about it and said, "I'm going to try it."

He came in for his appointment the following week and said, "I won't need you anymore after today."

I said, "Why not?"

He replied, "I've made love to this lovely lady three times this week and everything is perfect."

I said, "Tell me what happened."

He answered, "Well, I followed your advice and when things got to that certain place I said, 'I've got a problem and I want you to know this because it doesn't mean that you're...' everything you told me to say. She smiled and said, 'Honey, don't worry about that. You just leave everything to me.'" He said, "You know, it was just like magic."

Now in that case the therapeutic solution was that she took all the responsibility and fear away from him. She said in effect, "I'll take the responsibility. You needn't be concerned about anything." The moment that he didn't have to be anxious about performance or "satisfying her," his normal, natural function was restored and he never did have to come back to me for further therapy.

How did that relate to this problem with the spelling? The moment that you can be at that place where you know that you can spell and you have that experience of spelling, then you no longer have to have those expectations. You see, they're like shadows that are familiar to you, and when you look at the shadows, you feel the anxiety.

SCOTTY: Uh-huh.

BOYNE: The shadows are your fears about spelling.

SCOTTY: Right.

BOYNE: Quite often in dealing with a problem like this, a lot of other related content emerges. I'm about to hypnotize you now. Is there anything else you want to talk about or tell me or any other areas to investigate?

SCOTTY: No.

BOYNE: All right.

(BOYNE ADDRESSES THE AUDIENCE)

BOYNE: Earlier I made a comment. I said, "Store those things because that's something we're going to look for." Scotty said, "There is a trigger which allows me…" Finish it, Scotty.

SCOTTY: To spell perfectly.

BOYNE: Fine. Come right over here. Just pull your feet together. Just look at me. Take a deep breath and SLEEP NOW! (Boyne snaps his fingers as he says this and places his hand on Scotty's forehead) That's it. Relax all over now. Let every muscle and every nerve grow loose and limp and relaxed. All right. (Boyne rocks Scotty's head as he says this) Relax all over, every muscle and every nerve loose, limp, relaxed, and feel good now. That's fine. Now I'm going to lower you down to the floor, and as I do, just go much deeper in sleep. Here we go. Five, four, three, two, one. Now just sleep deeply. (Boyne has placed Scotty on the floor.) That's good. All right. That's fine.

INTENSIFYING THE PREDOMINANT SUBCONSCIOUS FEELING

Now there is the feeling that has to do with the trigger, the trigger that enables you to have that good feeling in which you know that you're able to spell. I'm going to count now from one up to ten and as I do, I want you to get in touch with that feeling. One, two, three, now the feeling begins to emerge. Four, five, six, it's a feeling of that trigger coming upon you. Six, seven, eight, nine, growing stronger and stronger now. (Boyne places his hand on Scotty's forehead as he says) Ten.

Now become aware of that feeling and the first thing is, I want you to tell me where in the body you feel it. Where does it seem to be centered in your body?

SCOTTY: It's centered in my upper body, in my stomach, and my chest and my arms.

BOYNE: Now give a description to the feeling. "It feels like…" or "it feels as if…."

SCOTTY: I'm confident.

BOYNE: Ah-ha! "I feel confident." Could you give a symbolic description to it? "I feel confident" is an interpretation of the feeling. I want you to create a symbol. If I felt very sad I might say, "My stomach feels like there is a heavy rock in it." Give me a symbolic description about this feeling that is like, "It feels like…" or, "it feels as if…."

SCOTTY: I feel strong.

BOYNE: "I feel strong." Say that again.

SCOTTY: I feel strong.

BOYNE: Again.

SCOTTY: I feel strong.

AGE REGRESSION

BOYNE: Now I'm going to count from ten down to one, and we're going back to a time when you are younger and it has to do with your strengths, feeling strong, feeling competent, feeling capable. Ten, nine, eight, you're drifting back. Seven, six, five, growing younger now. Four, your arms and legs are shrinking and you're growing smaller. Three, two, one. (Boyne places his hand on Scotty's forehead.) All right. Where you are, are you indoors or outside? (Boyne taps Scotty's forehead as he says) Quickly now make a choice. Pick one.

SCOTTY: I'm outside (in a childlike voice).

BOYNE: Outside. Daytime or nighttime?

SCOTTY: Daytime.

BOYNE: Alone or is someone with you or around you?

SCOTTY: With someone.

BOYNE: Who is it you're with?

SCOTTY: I'm with my friends.

BOYNE: Say it again.

SCOTTY: I'm with my friends.

BOYNE: Your friends. How old are you?

SCOTTY: Ten.

BOYNE: Ten years old. Give a report on what's going on?

SCOTTY: We're in the woods.

BOYNE: How do you feel there in the woods?

SCOTTY: Good.

BOYNE: Do you like being in the woods?

SCOTTY: Yes.

BOYNE: What's happening?

SCOTTY: We're running.

BOYNE: That's a good feeling to run in the woods; isn't it?

SCOTTY: Yes.

BOYNE: All right. Are you a fast runner?

SCOTTY: I can run further and faster than they can.

BOYNE: That's good. All right. Now you're running. What do you feel as you run?

SCOTTY: Free.

BOYNE: It's a feeling of freedom. And now what's happening?

SCOTTY: We're coming to town—we're getting closer to home.

BOYNE: As you get closer to home, tell me about your feeling. Is it the same?

SCOTTY: No.

BOYNE: How is it different?

SCOTTY: I don't feel free. I don't feel strong when I'm at home.

SIGNIFICANT STATEMENT

BOYNE: All right. Now I'm going to count from three down to one. You're going into the home, a situation in which you no longer feel free. You no longer feel strong, but rather you feel restricted and weak. All right. Three, two, one. (Boyne taps Scotty's forehead as he says) Where are you now?

SCOTTY: I'm inside.

BOYNE: All right. Are you alone or is someone with you?

SCOTTY: I'm with my grandmother.

BOYNE: With your grandmother. Do you love your grandmother?

SCOTTY: I don't like her.

BOYNE: Does she love you?

SCOTTY: Yes.

BOYNE: What is it about your grandmother that she does or doesn't do that makes you feel you don't like her?

SCOTTY: I—sometimes I don't like her.

BOYNE: All right. Tell me about those times. What is it she does at those times that makes you not like her?

SCOTTY: She is very mean.

BOYNE: She's mean. Can you tell me, "I don't like her when..." and then go on from there?

SCOTTY: I don't like her when she hits me.

BOYNE: Where does she hit you and for what reason?

SCOTTY: She hits me on the legs and the back.

BOYNE: All right. When I count to three, you go to a place where she's hitting you. One, two, three. (Boyne taps Scotty's forehead.) Now, feel her hitting you. (Boyne taps Scotty's legs.) How do you feel?

SCOTTY: I feel bad.

BOYNE: Can you tell me what the bad feeling is like?

SCOTTY: She beats me.

BOYNE: How old are you?

SCOTTY: Ten.

BOYNE: Are you a bad boy?

SCOTTY: Sometimes.

BOYNE: What do you do that's bad?

SCOTTY: I run away.

BOYNE: You run away. Do you live with your grandmother?

SCOTTY: Sometimes.

BOYNE: Sometimes, and the other times who do you live with?

SCOTTY: My mom and dad.

BOYNE: I see. Do you run away only from your grandmother or do you also run away when you're home with Mom and Dad?

SCOTTY: When I'm home.

BOYNE: When you're home you run away?

SCOTTY: Yes.

BOYNE: You don't run away from grandmother?

SCOTTY: I run away from grandmother.

BOYNE: You run away from both places?

SCOTTY: Yes.

BOYNE: All right. When you run away, where do you go?

SCOTTY: I go to the woods or to the creek.

BOYNE: And how do you feel when you're in the woods and at the creek?

SCOTTY: Free.

BOYNE: (Boyne places his hand on Scotty's forehead and says) Let your mind grow clear.

(BOYNE ADDRESSES THE AUDIENCE)

BOYNE: See, now we've isolated a very important kind of feeling, the feeling of freedom. That's his key. He has to feel free in order to have optimum function. Since feeling free is very subjective, we've got to do more work on him. We've got to uncover a great deal more, but we do have some important information: "I'm very functional when I feel free."

(BOYNE ADDRESSES SCOTTY)

BOYNE: When I count from three down to one, now you'll be seated in a chair and your grandmother is seated out in a chair in front of you. Three, two, one. There's your grandmother. I want you to talk to her and tell her how you feel. What do you call her—Grandma, Granny, Nanny? What do you call her?

SCOTTY: Grandma.

BOYNE: Grandma. Say, "Grandma, I want to tell you how I feel."

SCOTTY: Grandma, I want to tell you how I feel.

GESTALT DIALOGUE

BOYNE: Would you tell her now.

SCOTTY: When you hit me, I get very angry at you. And the day you beat me was the *first time anybody ever made me give up* and I don't like you.

SIGNIFICANT STATEMENT
FEELING OF HELPLESSNESS

BOYNE: Say that again.

SCOTTY: I don't like you.

BOYNE: Again.

SCOTTY: I don't like you.

BOYNE: Start it with, "The day you beat me..."

SCOTTY: The day you beat me, you made me give up and I don't like you.

SIGNIFICANT STATEMENT

BOYNE: Be the grandmother. Answer your grandson.

SCOTTY: (As the grandmother) Well, you had it coming.

BOYNE: Tell him why.

SCOTTY: (As the grandmother) You were wading in the creek and it was overflowing, and you could have been drowned. You made me angry and I beat you.

BOYNE: Now tell your grandson about how you were frightened for his safety before you got angry.

SCOTTY: Before I was angry at you, I was worried to death.

BOYNE: You worried about him, because of the way you feel toward him?

SCOTTY: (As the grandmother) Yes. He's a good boy, but he runs away a lot.

BOYNE: Tell him that. Tell him that.

SCOTTY: (As the grandmother) You're a good boy. You're a good boy.

BOYNE: Be the boy. Answer your grandmother.

SCOTTY: *That's the first time you've ever told me that and I believed it.*

CHANGING THE SUBCONSCIOUS FEELING

I hear you say I'm a good boy, but you always want me to do something when you call me a good boy.

BOYNE: Be the grandmother.

SCOTTY: (As the grandmother) Well, I don't understand what you mean. You're a good boy.

BOYNE: Do you love your grandson?

SCOTTY: (As the grandmother) Certainly I love my grandson.

BOYNE: Tell him that.

SCOTTY: (As the grandmother) I love you.

BOYNE: Be the boy.

SCOTTY: Well, I—I—I know you love me, but you want me to do things I don't want to do and first you call me a good boy so I go do it and if I don't do it then you beat me. You just want me to do what *you* want me to do.

CONDITIONAL LOVE

BOYNE: Make the statement, "I feel I'm only a good boy if I do what you want me to do."

SCOTTY: I feel I'm only a good boy if I do what you want me to do.

BOYNE: Be the grandmother.

SCOTTY: (As the grandmother) Well, that's right. I know what's good for you.

BOYNE: Be the boy.

SCOTTY: I don't care what you think about what's good for me. I want to do what I want to do.

EXPRESSION OF NEED FOR AUTONOMY

BOYNE: Say that again.

SCOTTY: I want to do what I want to do.

BOYNE: Again.

SCOTTY: I want to do what I want to do.

BOYNE: Be the grandmother.

SCOTTY: (As the grandmother) Yeah, and you always want to run away.

BOYNE: Be the boy.

SCOTTY: That's right. I want to run away. I don't like to be in the house all the time.

BOYNE: If you'll tell your grandmother how you feel in the woods and the creek, maybe that will help. Tell her, "When I run away and go down to the woods..." Tell her how you feel.

SCOTTY: When I go with the gang in the woods I feel—I feel great. I can run faster and we like each other, and I feel strong. I really feel good and I'm not afraid.

I FEEL COMPETENT AND ACCEPTED AND APPROVED

BOYNE: Say that again.

SCOTTY: And I'm not afraid.

BOYNE: Be the grandmother.

SCOTTY: (As the grandmother) Well, I'm afraid you'll hurt yourself. Why don't you stay home?

BOYNE: Be the boy.

SCOTTY: Well, I'm not going to stay home.

BOYNE: Say it again.

SCOTTY: I'm not going to stay home.

BOYNE: Again.

SCOTTY: I'm not going to stay home, and whatever you do, you can't keep me home all the time.

ASSERTION EXPRESSED AS DEFIANCE

BOYNE: All right, be the grandmother.

SCOTTY: (As the grandmother) Well, I don't mean all the time, but just stay close.

BOYNE: Be the boy.

SCOTTY: No. I'm ten years old. I'm not going to stick around like a *sissy*. I feel good with the gang. I feel good. I'm going to do what I'm going to do.

LACK OF MALE ROLE MODEL—NO MENTION OF FATHER AS YET!

BOYNE: Say that again.

SCOTTY: I'm going to do what I want to do.

BOYNE: Again.

SCOTTY: I'm going to do what I want to do.

BOYNE: Let your mind grow clear. (Camera fades to black and fades up again. Scotty is lying on a couch.) When I count to three, I want you to raise your leg up in the air. (Boyne lifts Scotty's legs in demonstration.) Kick it into the couch. Then the other leg—kick it into the couch. Continue kicking alternately until I tell you to stop. One, two, three. Begin. (Scotty is kicking.) That's it. Kick it down hard. Each time you kick it down, say the word *no*.

SCOTTY: No. No.

BOYNE: Louder.

SCOTTY: NO!

BOYNE: Do as you are told.

SCOTTY: NO!

BOYNE: Give in.

SCOTTY: NO!

BOYNE: Listen to your grandmother.

SCOTTY: NO!

BOYNE: Be a good boy.

SCOTTY: NO!

BOYNE: Stay out of the woods.

SCOTTY: NO!

BOYNE: Do as you're told.

SCOTTY: NO!

BOYNE: Be nice.

SCOTTY: NO!

BOYNE: Say, "No I won't." Keep kicking. Say, "No I won't."

SCOTTY: No.

BOYNE: "No I won't."

SCOTTY: No I won't.

BOYNE: Louder.

SCOTTY: NO I WON'T!

BOYNE: Shout it.

SCOTTY: (Shouting) NO I WON'T!

BOYNE: That's good. Keep kicking.

SCOTTY: (Shouting) NO I WON'T!

BOYNE: Listen to your mother.

SCOTTY: (Shouting) NO I WON'T!

BOYNE: Be a good boy.

SCOTTY: NO I WON'T!

BOYNE: Give in.

SCOTTY: NO I WON'T!

BOYNE: Yes you will.

SCOTTY: NO I WON'T!

BOYNE: You'll do it now.

SCOTTY: (Shouting) NO I WON'T!

BOYNE: Oh, yes you will.

SCOTTY: (Shouting) NO I WON'T!

BOYNE: You've got to now.

SCOTTY: (Shouting) NO I WON'T!

BOYNE: Rest. Go into and go through your body and become aware of whatever you are experiencing—feelings, sensations, lack of feeling, lack of sensation, numbness. Go from the top of your head to the tip of your toes and then give a report.

SCOTTY: My chest and my arms feel strong.

BOYNE: "My chest and my arms feel strong." What about the lower half of the body? What do you feel in the pelvis, the legs?

SCOTTY: I feel mostly my feet, my heels. I feel the pressure.

BOYNE: What are you experiencing in your pelvis, stomach, abdomen?

SCOTTY: I feel strong.

BOYNE: When I touch your forehead, I want you to start kicking again. (Boyne taps Scotty's forehead and says) All right, begin. Each time you kick say, "I resent you."

SCOTTY: I resent you. I resent you.

BOYNE: Louder.

SCOTTY: I resent you.

BOYNE: Shout it.

SCOTTY: (Shouting) I RESENT YOU!

BOYNE: Louder.

SCOTTY: I RESENT YOU!

BOYNE: Shout it.

SCOTTY: (Shouting) I RESENT YOU!

BOYNE: Say, "You scare me."

SCOTTY: (Silence)

BOYNE: "I resent you."

SCOTTY: I resent you.

BOYNE: Keep kicking until I tell you to stop. "I resent you."

SCOTTY: I resent you.

BOYNE: Louder.

SCOTTY: I RESENT YOU!

BOYNE: Say, "You scare me."

SCOTTY: No.

BOYNE: Say it.

SCOTTY: No.

PHOBIC AVOIDANCE OF ACKNOWLEDGING FEAR

BOYNE: Say it now.

SCOTTY: (Screaming) NO!

BOYNE: Say it now!

SCOTTY: (Screaming) NO!

BOYNE: (Boyne places his hand on Scotty's forehead and says) Rest. Tend to your breathing now. At the same time take your mind, go into and go all through your body, become aware of the experiences, feeling, sensation, lack of sensation.

SCOTTY: My hands feel heavy.

BOYNE: All right, what else?

SCOTTY: I feel strong. My stomach is tight.

BOYNE: Can you describe it? "It feels like…," "It feels as if…."

SCOTTY: It feels like I want to hit.

BOYNE: Where in your stomach is that feeling that you want to hit?

SCOTTY: My arms.

BOYNE: All right.

SCOTTY: My stomach is tight.

BOYNE: Tight. Give that a description. "My stomach is tight and it feels as if…, it feels like…."

SCOTTY: I'm holding tight so if I get hit, I won't get the wind knocked out of me.

BOYNE: All right. (Boyne taps Scotty's forehead as he says) Start kicking again. Say, "Leave me alone."

SCOTTY: Leave me alone.

BOYNE: Louder.

SCOTTY: Leave me alone.

BOYNE: Shout it!

SCOTTY: (Shouting) LEAVE ME ALONE! LEAVE ME ALONE!

BOYNE: All right. Go into your throat and become aware of what you're experiencing.

SCOTTY: It's burning.

BOYNE: Describe the sensation in your throat.

SCOTTY: It's scratchy.

BOYNE: Anything else?

SCOTTY: Kind of closed.

BOYNE: It seems as if you started to choke back some of that energy.

SCOTTY: Yeah.

BOYNE: (Boyne places Scotty's hand around his forearm as he says) I want to bring your other hand up. Bring this hand up and take hold now. All right. I want you to begin to squeeze my arm when I count to three. One, two, three. Now as you do, I want you to say, "I'll choke you."

SCOTTY: I'll choke you.

BOYNE: Do it now.

SCOTTY: (Scotty has both his hands around Gil's arm as he says) I'll choke you.

BOYNE: "I'll kill you."

SCOTTY: I SAID I'll KILL YOU!

BOYNE: Do it.

SCOTTY: I'll KILL YOU!

BOYNE: Shout it!

SCOTTY: (Shouting) I'll KILL YOU! I'll KILL YOU! I'll KILL YOU! I'll KILL YOU!

BOYNE: Open your throat.

SCOTTY: (Shouting) I'll KILL YOU!

BOYNE: Open it now.

SCOTTY: I'll KILL YOU!

BOYNE: (Boyne places his hand on Scotty's forehead and says) Rest. Rest. Tend to your breathing now. (Boyne places his hand on Scotty's stomach, chest, legs.) All right. Go into your body now and give a report.

SCOTTY: My arms are tired.

BOYNE: Your throat?

SCOTTY: It's still scratchy, but it's not closed.

BOYNE: You no longer have to choke yourself.

SCOTTY: No, I feel strength in my legs. They feel good.

BOYNE: Now just relax and let your mind grow clear.

(BOYNE ADDRESSES THE AUDIENCE)

BOYNE: Now he's starting to get grounded. That's the first time he reported strength in the legs. We're starting to put a support under him and ground him.

(BOYNE ADDRESSES SCOTTY)

BOYNE: Okay. What else is going on? Talk about your feelings. Any ideas flashing? Any feelings when you were expressing some of those phrases?

SCOTTY: I don't know who I want to kill. I don't want to kill my grandmother or my parents. I don't know who I want to kill.

BOYNE: Okay. Start kicking again. Get the legs up. Kick hard now. Say, "I hate you."

SCOTTY: I hate you.

BOYNE: Louder.

SCOTTY: I HATE YOU!

BOYNE: Louder.

SCOTTY: I HATE YOU!

BOYNE: Shout it!

SCOTTY: (Shouting) I HATE YOU! I HATE YOU!

BOYNE: Again.

SCOTTY: I HATE YOU!

BOYNE: Again.

SCOTTY: I HATE YOU!

BOYNE: Again.

SCOTTY: Hate you (softer).

BOYNE: Again.

SCOTTY: Hate you (softer).

BOYNE: (Whispers) Say, "And I love you."

SCOTTY: I love you.

BOYNE: Again.

SCOTTY: I love you.

BOYNE: Again.

SCOTTY: (Soft crying)

BOYNE: (Pause) All right. Go into your body now and give a report.

SCOTTY: (He sits up.)

BOYNE: Slide down a little bit on the couch. Push your body down a little bit.

SCOTTY: (He moves his body down.)

BOYNE: That's it. Now sleep deeply. Go deeper now. It's all right. (Boyne rocks Scotty's forehead as he says) That's it. All right. What's going on now?

SCOTTY: I—whatever it is I feel I want to kill, I love it just as much. I want to cry.

AMBIVALENT FEELINGS

BOYNE: Can you stay with that feeling—wanting to cry?

SCOTTY: Okay.

BOYNE: I want you to raise both arms. (Boyne takes Scotty's arm and holds it up in demonstration.) Hold them out like that. Now I'll give you a choice. I want you to call for your grandma or your ma or your father, whichever one of the three you want to call for. Who would you like to call for?

SCOTTY: *My father.*

UNMENTIONED UNTIL NOW

BOYNE: All right. Call for him. What do you call him, Dad?

SCOTTY: Yeah.

BOYNE: "Dad, where are you?"

SCOTTY: Dad, where are you?

BOYNE: Call again.

SCOTTY: Dad, Daddy.

BOYNE: Call for him again.

SCOTTY: Daddy.

BOYNE: Can you say, "I need you, Daddy"?

SCOTTY: I need you.

BOYNE: Again.

SCOTTY: I need you, Daddy.

BOYNE: Here's what I want you to do. I want you to make a statement. Say, "I'm a good boy, Daddy." Start with that, "I'm a good boy, Daddy."

SCOTTY: I'm a good boy, Daddy.

BOYNE: "Daddy, when I grow up...." Tell him that.

SCOTTY: Daddy, when I grow up.

BOYNE: Tell him what you're going to do or be when you grow up. "When I grow up…"

SCOTTY: When I grow up, I want to be just like you (crying).

BOYNE: All right. Start again. "When I grow up…" Finish it in a new way. "When I grow up…"

SCOTTY: Daddy, when I grow up, I want to treat my kids better than you treat me (harder crying).

BOYNE: Start again. Finish it in a new way.

SCOTTY: Daddy, when I grow up, I'm never going away from my kids.

BOYNE: Start again. "When I grow up…"

SCOTTY: When I grow up, I'm going to love my kids.

BOYNE: Start again.

SCOTTY: When I grow up, I'm never going to leave them (harder crying).

INTERPRETATION: "WHEN YOU LEFT US, I FELT ABANDONED AND UNLOVED."

BOYNE: All right. Again.

SCOTTY: Daddy, when I grow up, I'm not going to be as mean as you are.

BOYNE: Again.

SCOTTY: Daddy, when I grow up, I'm never going to leave my kids.

BOYNE: Drop your arms. Now listen carefully. This time when you start kicking I want you to bring all those promises back. It goes like this as you kick. You say, "No, I don't have to be like you. No, I can leave my kids if I want to," and so on. Reverse all the promises that you made. All right. One, two, three. Begin. "I don't have to be like you."

SCOTTY: I don't have to be like you.

BOYNE: Again.

SCOTTY: I can leave my kids if I want to.

BOYNE: Louder.

SCOTTY: I can leave my kids if I want to.

BOYNE: Louder.

SCOTTY: I can leave my kids if I want to. I can do any damn thing I want to.

BOYNE: Again.

SCOTTY: (Shouting) I CAN DO ANY DAMN THING I WANT TO!

BOYNE: "I'll do what I want to do."

SCOTTY: I'LL DO WHAT I WANT TO DO!

BOYNE: Kick faster.

SCOTTY: I'LL DO WHAT I WANT TO DO!

BOYNE: Hit with your fists. Go crazy.

SCOTTY: (Scotty is shouting, kicking, and pounding his fists down on the couch as he says) I'LL DO WHAT I WANT TO!

BOYNE: That's it, go crazy!

SCOTTY: Do what I want to do (softer, but defiant).

BOYNE: Do all that you want to do now.

SCOTTY: I'm going to do it (assertively).

BOYNE: All right.

SCOTTY: (Shouting and kicking) I'M DOING IT. I'M GOING TO DO IT!

BOYNE: Rest now. (Boyne places his hand on Scotty's forehead and rocks his head.) Go into your body. Become aware of what you're experiencing.

SCOTTY: I feel my arms and I feel my legs. I feel the blood going through my body.

BOYNE: You're aware that's the first time you said that that you felt the blood going through your body. Are you saying you feel more alive?

SCOTTY: I feel more alive, yes. I feel strong. I feel my arms tingling.

BOYNE: Now you remember that feeling of freedom?

SCOTTY: Yeah.

BOYNE: All right. We're going to move toward it right now. Raise your foot there. Raise the other one there. (Boyne has Scotty raise his feet so that his knees are bent and his feet are flat on the mattress.) Here's what I want you to do. Put the palms of your hands there. When I count to three, you'll raise your pelvis up and bring it down. (Boyne lifts Scotty's pelvis in demonstration of Pelvic Banging.) Let it bang like this and bounce and bang as high as you can. All right. One, two, three. Begin. All right. Say, "I'm free."

SCOTTY: I'm free.

BOYNE: Louder.

SCOTTY: FREE.

BOYNE: Louder.

SCOTTY: I'm FREE.

BOYNE: Just the word *free*.

SCOTTY: FREE.

BOYNE: Shout it!

SCOTTY: (Shouting) FREE!

BOYNE: Louder!

SCOTTY: FREE!

BOYNE: Go higher.

SCOTTY: FREE. (Scotty arches his back and locks his body in the arched position.)

BOYNE: Rest. Stay with the feeling. (Scotty falls back on the couch.)

SCOTTY: Oh, my arms, my back, oh.

BOYNE: What's the feeling?

SCOTTY: It's cramped. It hurts.

BOYNE: Can you turn it loose now? Are you ready to?

SCOTTY: Yeah. I want to turn it loose.

BOYNE: As I count to three, I want you to clench your fists and draw your whole body up tight and when I reach number three, we're going to turn it all loose. One, start clenching. Two, pull it all up tight. Three. (Boyne places his hand on Scotty's forehead and says) Turn it all loose.

SCOTTY: (Explosive screaming sound)

BOYNE: That's right. Now you can relax. Go into your body and through it and give a report.

SCOTTY: I can still feel the pain in both my arms.

BOYNE: All right.

SCOTTY: My back feels like it's cramped and my hands are numb.

BOYNE: Your hands are numb. What do you experience in your chest?

SCOTTY: Tight.

BOYNE: All right. Now I want you to become aware of what happens as you make an effort to move to freedom, to feel freedom, to become free. I want you to be aware of your phobic avoidance of acknowledging fear, your refusal to say, "You scare me." I want you to take as much time as you need to analyze it. Find out how those programmed responses link in with your avoidance of spelling. Take the time you need to think about it, and when you're ready to talk about it, just begin. Three, two, one. Now look back and analyze it.

SCOTTY: My acceptance of fear.

BOYNE: Open that up. What does it mean?

SCOTTY: If I accept the fear, I'll feel helpless.

BOYNE: "If I acknowledge the fear, I feel helpless." Now what do you do to keep from acknowledging the feeling of fear at times? How do you avoid that?

SCOTTY: I don't breathe.

BOYNE: "I restrict my breathing." That's true because all feelings require oxygen to be experienced and we tend to inhibit many kinds of strong feelings. Many people don't fully enjoy their sexual function because as the feelings become more and more intense, they restrict their breathing. All right. How does this relate to your behavior about spelling?

SCOTTY: When I feel free and strong, I don't care what people think about my spelling.

BOYNE: Now I have a question to ask you. Do you have a belief in some creative force outside yourself or, if not, perhaps a belief in your fellow man?

SCOTTY: I believe in a creative force outside myself.

BOYNE: If you believe in a creative force, then that is your symbol for God; is that right?

SCOTTY: That's right.

BOYNE: When you are paralyzed by constantly projecting out critical thoughts into the minds of others, you're worshipping the god of "what will people think," aren't you?

SCOTTY: Yes.

BOYNE: That's a pretty stupid god. You know, we can laugh at primitive religions that make gods of cats and turtles and frogs and all kinds of things, but we do the same thing when we worship the god of "what will people think about my behavior."

SCOTTY: Yeah.

BOYNE: What do you think you'd like to do so that you can come to an appropriate belief; a belief for an intelligent, mature, educated man of wisdom; a belief that's appropriate for you—a strong man, a courageous man, a free man?

SCOTTY: I believe if I get myself out of the way that God will flow through me.

BOYNE: Talk about it in terms of behavior.

SCOTTY: If I am unafraid of whatever people think, I can do my best.

BOYNE: (Boyne places his hand on Scotty's forehead and says) Let your mind grow clear now for a moment or two. (Boyne takes hold of Scotty's hand and says) Now in a moment I'm going to get you up. Before I do, is there anything further that you want to say to me or ask me or tell me?

SCOTTY: I want a word that I can say to myself to remind me I can spell perfectly.

BOYNE: That word is within you. I'm going to tap your forehead three times. The word will come to you. Ready? (Boyne taps Scotty's forehead three times.)

SCOTTY: Perfect.

BOYNE: Then that's your symbol. Quickly now, who do I remind you of?

SCOTTY: My uncle.

BOYNE: How am I like your uncle?

SCOTTY: We were friends. He was good to me.

BOYNE: That's good. I'm going to count from one to five. At the count of five, eyelids open, feeling good. One, slowly, calmly, easily, and gently returning to your full awareness once again. Two, each muscle and nerve in your body is loose and limp and relaxed, and you feel wonderfully good. Three, from head to toe you're feeling perfect in every way. Number four, you're eyes begin to feel sparkling clear. On the next number now, eyelids open, fully aware, feeling good in every way. Number five, let them open now. Take a deep breath. Fill up your lungs and stretch. All right, when you're ready, I want you to stand up and face the group now.

SCOTTY: (He stands up and faces the audience.)

BOYNE: Stand here with me. Let's start with that man. Can you say to him, "From now on I'm going to try to see the person you are instead of projecting my images of critical thoughts of me onto you. I'm going to stop using you and see you." Say something like that to him in your own words.

SCOTTY: I'm not going to see you as anything but what you are—a human being just like me.

BOYNE: Good. Give the next man an existential message about what happens if you read some disapproval coming from him.

SCOTTY: If you disapprove of me and I don't like it, you'll know it.

BOYNE: Good. Tell the next man something.

SCOTTY: If I like you, you'll know it.

BOYNE: Good. Tell Peter something.

SCOTTY: If I want to be your friend, you'll know it.

BOYNE: Talk to Jack.

SCOTTY: I'm not going to hide my feelings anymore.

BOYNE: Good. Now the lady.

SCOTTY: (Smiles) I want you to know I feel free.

BOYNE: And Joe.

SCOTTY: I'm very happy to know you.

BOYNE: Good. Now come on back up here. Let's sum up. Can you tell me where you are and what the feeling is and how you feel about this experience?

SCOTTY: I felt very comfortable. One of the things that I had been thinking about with my spelling difficulty was that I was afraid to spell, and I would not accept the fear of it—but this experience has shown me that I have been kidding myself about my fear and telling myself I had accepted all my fear when I was nowhere close.

BOYNE: You saw how difficult it was even to say here, "You scare me."

SCOTTY: That's right.

BOYNE: "I resent you" and "you scare me" are really the same statement, aren't they?

SCOTTY: That's right.

BOYNE: Or correlative statements, because we resent anything or anyone that produces fear in us.

SCOTTY: Uh-huh.

BOYNE: So when you project out, "He's thinking critical thoughts of me; I can tell by Peter's face he's thinking a critical thought of me. What right has he got to think that rotten thought about me?" the resentment and the fear, "You scare me," go together, especially in the child.

SCOTTY: (He nods in agreement).

BOYNE: That's what we're dealing with in this infantile protest and the release of locked-up energies. Now are you aware, when you made the move toward the feeling of freedom, how you locked up your back and your legs?

SCOTTY: Yes.

BOYNE: That's interesting, isn't it.

SCOTTY: (He nods in agreement.)

BOYNE: What's the message?

SCOTTY: That it's still locked.

BOYNE: You discovered how you do it. We don't need too much emphasis on why. Maybe you did get some whys, but you discovered what you do and how you do it. You discover how you choke yourself.

SCOTTY: Uh-huh.

BOYNE: The moment you did unto others as you do unto yourself and you choked my wrist, your throat opened up.

SCOTTY: (He nods in agreement.)

BOYNE: You did a lot of good work tonight, and I'm very pleased with you and what happened. (Boyne hugs Scotty and says) And I'm happy that you think of me like your uncle and feel that I'm good to you. I like being good to people. It feels good.

AUDIENCE: (Applause.)

END OF SESSION THREE.

THE CASE OF SCOTTY
The World's Worst Speller
Follow-up

(The Setting: A Classroom)

(BOYNE ADDRESSES THE AUDIENCE)

BOYNE: This is Gil Boyne and I'm pleased to tell you that I have Scotty with me here and this is June 1982, just five years since we last worked together.

(BOYNE ADDRESSES SCOTTY)

Scotty, delighted to have you back.

SCOTTY: Thank you.

BOYNE: Now you've just seen the film again after five years— give me a report! Tell me about your thoughts and feelings and your development since then.

SCOTTY: Well, the feelings as I watched it again were pretty strong feelings, but it seems as though a lot of the emotion, the energy of it has gone away. It's not there anymore. I have worked through it and my feeling is that there has been a distinct change in many of my habits.

BOYNE: That's a good word, *habits.*

SCOTTY: Yes! And I just get better. It's not finished, but I don't have to devote as much energy to the negative form as I had in the past.

BOYNE: You no longer mobilize and use your energy non-productively in being concerned and anxious about spelling and how other people will be concerned whether or not you spell the word correctly.

SCOTTY: Right, that gets less and less. As I said before, I started to write and have been involved in some scripts and I think that's a big step.

BOYNE: I understand you are working on a screenplay right now.

SCOTTY: Yes, I've decided to do one by myself.

BOYNE: I think that you mentioned the realization has come to you that even if you misspell a word, there are secretaries whose job it is to correct the spelling when they type.

SCOTTY: That's right.

BOYNE: You said "unfinished." I got the feeling earlier in talking to you that you've come to the position that life itself is a therapy and that you're constantly moving, growing, and expanding.

SCOTTY: That's the way I feel about it. It's a continuing experience. There might be a little time when you get a rest, so to speak. Or you have other things in front of you that you don't have the time to work on yourself, but when the dust settles, it's always there for the asking.

BOYNE: I know you're in the people-helping field.

SCOTTY: (He nods in agreement.)

BOYNE: I understand you are currently working in a hospital, is that right?

SCOTTY: Yes.

BOYNE: What department do you work in?

SCOTTY: I work in a chemical dependency center.

BOYNE: That is great work.

SCOTTY: I've been there for six years. It's a very good unit.

BOYNE: That's work that is satisfying to you.

SCOTTY: Yes. There's a tremendous amount of satisfaction in it, although it holds its frustrations.

BOYNE: Yes, the addictive personality is a frustrating one to deal with. My father was an addictive personality, an alcoholic. I think that predisposes me in my reactions and prevents me from being most effective in working with alcoholics. But I'm happy there are people like you that I can refer them to.

SCOTTY: My father was an alcoholic also. He was able to effectively stop drinking when he was around thirty-five years old, and I found that the situation that I grew up with had a lot to do with what happened. I find many people that I work with had the same background.

BOYNE: In the exciting therapy we filmed, some of the energy that you expressed was directed toward your internalized images of your father and mother. Did that lead to any connection, any contact with either of your parents afterwards?

SCOTTY: Well, my father was deceased at that point. I had always been in contact with my mother and it had been a difficult relationship for many years. Although I didn't really make it difficult for her, I kept a lot of that feeling to myself, but she was diagnosed with terminal cancer about two years ago and died on Christmas. There was a year and a half when I was given the opportunity to really finish up with my mother and close the book.

BOYNE: And take care of unfinished business.

SCOTTY: That's right, and it was really good. It was a real good situation and I was able to forgive and forget, and I mean really forget it, not the self-righteous forgiveness.

BOYNE: The best forgiveness is when you do forget.

SCOTTY: Amen!

BOYNE: Well, Scotty, you were just inside a few moments ago in our classroom, and after everyone saw the film, they all felt that you are really transformed. You seem to have so much more self-assurance—so much more internal togetherness that is radiating outward. I'm delighted to have you back here with us. Let's look forward to making more contact.

SCOTTY: Okay, that's great feedback from the students. The class was really great, felt good.

(BOYNE ADDRESSES THE AUDIENCE)

BOYNE: You know now that Scotty really wasn't the world's worst speller, although he clung to the title for years. Then he surrendered it, and now he's just one of the world's great human beings—at least in his own opinion, and that's where it really counts.

Until the next time, this is Gil Boyne.

HYPNOTHERAPY FOR OVERCOMING
PERFORMANCE ANXIETY

The Case of Pat ("Fear of Public Speaking")

A mature, intelligent female hypnotherapy student reports a fear of public speaking. She states that she "always sounds haughty" when speaking to a group.

A comprehensive intake interview fails to reveal any evidence of negative childhood experiences or identifications. Trance is induced and deepened and a highly specialized program of affirmations and visualizations is presented.

THE CASE OF PAT
"Fear of Public Speaking"

(BOYNE ADDRESSES AUDIENCE)

BOYNE: Hello. This is Gil Boyne. Welcome to the hypnotherapy video clinic. Today we're here with one of our students from the clinical hypnotherapy class; let's meet her now.

(BOYNE ADDRESSES PAT)

Pat, welcome. Since you have been in class, you have been seeing some case histories of people I've worked with, you've seen successful resolutions of problems, cure of various conditions, and you came up and asked if I would work with you for a specific response. What is it that you want help with?

PAT: I have a friend who belongs to a businesswomen's group, and she's asked me to see her when I get back. She was very nice. She said, "As soon as you're ready, let me know and you can talk to my group."

BOYNE: Have you ever done any speaking to groups?

PAT: Only very small groups, maybe four or five people, like to give a nursing report every shift so that I speak to a group at that point.

BOYNE: It's said that the most common fear is the fear of speaking in public, but there is no such thing as public speaking. If there were, there would have to be private speaking, and we do that all the time when we talk to ourselves. The fear is really a fear of speaking to groups. Everyone who reports this fear will say, "I don't have any fear when talking with one or two people." Essentially, the fear of public speaking is a fear of criticism or a symptom of the fear of criticism. In essence, the person is saying, "I can cope, I can manage, I can adjust and change if I feel some disapproval about what I'm saying, provided there are only one or two people present. When I'm standing in front of a group, I have no control and they're all going to think terrible, critical thoughts about me. They're going to notice mistakes I make," and so on. That's really the root of all that fear!

Here's how it developed. Back in the second grade, there was a time the teacher called on little Jimmy and she said, "Jimmy, spell cat." And Jimmy was so nervous, he went "ah, ah" and everyone laughed and Jimmy felt that it meant he was ridiculous. The other children laughed to relieve their tensions—they were so relieved that it wasn't them standing there. But from then on Jimmy holds that memory, and even makes a promise to himself: "I'll never get up in front of a group again and give them the opportunity to see me in a ridiculous situation and to laugh at me again and cause me to feel this humiliation." He may go through his whole lifetime and never speak to a group again. I know that seems oversimplified, but having done thousands of age regressions, I've found that occurring over and over again.

Are you aware of any fears speaking to groups?

PAT: I'm not aware of any particular fear. I also remembered another group. I was president of the parents' club at school, and I did talk to the parents. But in order for me to do that, I was very nervous and spoke haughtily as I do now. Also, I had to make myself very precise notes and stick to them on the lectern so that I could handle it. I did not feel like I made a good presentation.

BOYNE: You didn't feel you were as effective as you could be.

PAT: Exactly.

BOYNE: One of the things that is helpful as you review your material, instead of taking the notes and being confined to the reading of the notes, break it into short paragraphs and summarize those paragraphs with one or two or three words. Now you can make up a list with a marking pen and take it to the lectern, and you'll find that those few words will keep triggering off entire paragraphs. All you have to do is glance down and pick up your key words. You can even hold your hand up on the lectern and let your finger be a pointer as to where you are, and that will increase your spontaneity. To be tied to what is written down is not an effective way of speaking.

Many years ago, I used to teach self-hypnosis from a curriculum, and it got to the point that I had committed everything to memory after hundreds of repetitions. I got to feeling that I was simply a recording machine—I always told the same jokes at the same place and laughed at the same place and so on—and I was burning out. Then one day I said, "No, I'm going to rearrange this material. I'm going to teach it extemporaneously. I'm going to allow for me to shift part B up to where D normally is and so on. I'm going to allow for interaction with the group. Once I did that, I liberated myself and ever since then, even though I've taught clinical hypnotherapy to more than six thousand persons, I have never worked from a printed script again. I know what I have to teach and I know how I'm going to teach it, and yet I can make it fresh each time.

So you really don't have any bad experiences of panicking when you went to speak or not being able to sleep the night before or imagining a catastrophe in speaking or anything like that.

PAT: As you just said that, just one thing comes to mind. In my high school years I was in a small, little play. It was kind of like a drama class, and I thought I had memorized my lines very well, but when it came time to say them, I again had trouble saying them. It wasn't that I didn't say them.

BOYNE: You didn't freeze.

PAT: But it came out pretty haughtily, it didn't come out the way I wanted.

BOYNE: How did you feel at that time?

PAT: I would say a little panicked. I mean, I feel simply panicked right through so I don't feel like, like I feel, somewhat feeling right now in this, so, you know, it doesn't seem to be...

BOYNE: Are there any other areas in which you have the same kind of feelings, performance anxiety?

PAT: Exactly! I have performance anxiety. I can play the piano, easily, for my own pleasure. If I try to play something that I had played calmly, easily at home when there is someone who might try to sing or pay attention to me in some way, I would make many mistakes.

BOYNE: The fear of making the mistake produces mistakes, doesn't it?

PAT: I guess that's right, sure.

BOYNE: Job said in the old testament. "The things that I have feared have come upon me," which is a great psychological truth. It is called the rule of mental expectancy. "That which I fear has come upon me." What is expected tends to be realized. When we say, "I'm afraid. I don't want to make a mistake. I'm afraid I might make a mistake." That creates a mental image which acts as a blueprint and literally says to the subconscious, "Make a mistake."

PAT: Right.

BOYNE: And so you do. I once had a woman who suffered badly from performance anxiety, she had been a concert pianist and now she was the pianist for the L. A. Ballet Company, and although she had no problem in rehersals, on the night of the performance her fingers would grow so stiff that it interfered with her playing. It took a number of sessions before she could learn to relax. Because that's really what it was, tension anxiety. In two full weeks in this class, I guess you've seen I'm much the same when teaching as when I'm not teaching. I am as relaxed in front of the group as I am on the coffee break. Do you agree?

PAT: I agree to that.

BOYNE: Some just call it confidence, but I call it knowing that I can cope, knowing that I can manage a class with thirty or forty people in it and a business with five employees simultaneously and all the things that occur and all the demands on me. Of course, part of that is the experience of having done it for a very long period of time. Do you feel that performance anxiety is something that really overwhelms you?

PAT: I'd say that the degree is not particularly severe. If we were saying from one to ten, one being the worst and ten being the best, I'm probably a seven and a half.

BOYNE: So you don't have any real phobic avoidances. You don't break out in a sweat knowing that you have to give a talk, toss and turn the night before, or experience nausea fifteen minutes before you have to talk.

PAT: I remember for the parents' club meeting I did toss and turn the night before, but after several of them I did not continue to do that.

BOYNE: So you know the world is going to keep turning and you're going to wake up the next day even if you do make a mistake while speaking.

PAT: That's right, but I want to do a good job.

BOYNE: Sure you do. If you did a good job, would you then be glad or are you a perfectionist?

PAT: I'd be thrilled. I'd be thrilled. (You can see the rapport building between Gil and Pat.)

BOYNE: Be sure you don't set perfectionistic standards, "I have to be perfect so that no one can criticize me."

PAT: No, I just want the people to understand me and enjoy my presentation.

BOYNE: All right, fine.

PAT: That's really what I want.

BOYNE: Are you ready for me to hypnotize you?

PAT: Yes.

BOYNE: Good. Would you please push your chair back. Please separate your legs. All right, just rest your arms and your hands on the arms of the chair. Look at me. Take a deep breath now and fill up your lungs. Exhale slowly. Relax. Now a second and even deeper breath. Exhale. Relax. Now a third deep breath, and I'll count from five down to one. As I do, your eyelids grow heavy, droopy, drowsy, and sleepy. By the time I reach the count of one, they close right down. You go deep in hypnotic slumber.

Five, eyelids heavy, droopy, drowsy, and sleepy. Four, the next time they blink that's hypnosis coming on them. Three, your heavy lids close. Two, now they're closing even tighter. One, now just SLEEP! (Gil taps Pat's forehead.) And relax. Make no further effort as each muscle and nerve begins to grow loose and limp and relaxed. I'm going to count from ten down to one. With each number I count, you'll feel yourself drifting, relaxing, turning loose, and letting go. Ten, each muscle and nerve grows loose and limp and relaxed. Nine, you are relaxing more with each easy breath that you take. Eight, you're drifting down calmly, quietly, easily, and gently. Seven, six, go way down now. Five, when I reach the count of one, I'll say the words "sleep deeply." You'll then be aware you're more deeply relaxed than ever before. Four, drifting down. Three, two, on the next number I'll give the signal. Now get ready. Number one, now just sleep deeply. (Gil taps Pat's forehead lightly.)

I'm now going to give you some good, powerful, creative and positive suggestions. Each of these suggestions will make a very deep, vivid, and permanent impression on your subconscious mind. Don't try to think about the suggestions or list them, just let your mind drift where it will into hypnosis.

As you go deeper, you're becoming aware that you like people. You enjoy being with people. You are poised and confident when talking with good friends or new acquaintances. You are secure and relaxed when you are with people. You especially like speaking to people. People are aware that you like them, and they return the feeling. People like you. People like to listen to you. People enjoy your company. You are at ease when you are with people. When you stand before a group, you are filled with feelings of friendliness for them. You want to do things for them. You experience a feeling of warmth and friendship flowing from the members of the group to you. You have a feeling that they are on your side. You are interested in them. You want to do things for them. You feel a sense of personal friendship with every member of the audience.

As you speak, you are perfectly poised, self-possessed, and completely free in your expression. You feel at ease. You present your ideas in a clear, brief, and direct way, and your ideas are quickly understood and accepted by others. Your mind is clear. Your wit is quick. Your lips are flexible. Your mouth is moist. Your breathing is deep and from the diaphragm. Your hands are poised and calm. Your gestures flow spontaneously and freely. You speak easily, always giving a clear word picture of the thought you wish to convey. You're poised and in control of the situation. Your legs are strong beneath you. You are comfortable and peaceful. You are secure and confident as you speak. You speak spontaneously, sincerely, and freely; clearly expressing your meaning and feelings. At any time when you speak, whether to a large audience or a small group, as you begin you feel this warmth and friendliness for your listeners. As you begin, you feel their friendliness directed toward you. You are totally confident. You are perfectly at ease. As you begin to talk, you have the undivided attention of the audience and it makes you feel good. You speak freely, fluently, with a full release of your skill and your talent. You thoroughly enjoy speaking to an audience. Whenever you feel you can add a viewpoint or interesting facts to a discussion, you speak openly and confidently. You communicate effectively at all times. People seek your opinions on a variety of subjects, and you express information in an interesting and witty manner. You have a special talent for expressing your thoughts and ideas vividly with enthusiasm that impresses everyone who hears you.

When others speak, you listen and you learn from them. You see their point of view. You express your ideas in a positive way whenever possible. When you speak, your voice is strong, calm, and vibrant. Your lines flow with concise and yet powerful messages whenever you will them to do so. Your voice is pleasant to hear. People are eager to hear what you have to say because you are so alive and so vibrant. The friendship within you radiates outward to touch each person with whom you come in contact. You ask questions when you don't understand, and you state your opinions whenever you are asked. People respect your opinions because they recognize that they are honest and well thought out. You speak spontaneously, sincerely, and freely; clearly verbalizing your feelings. When there is nothing for you to say, you radiate interest, empathy, and concern. You are so interested in people, you stimulate them to express their views. When words are inadequate, you act out your feelings. When you are called upon to conduct a meeting, you are relaxed, in complete control of the situation. You are physically relaxed, with an inner calmness, a sense of well-being, a self-assurance. Your conversation is bright and informative. Your talent for expressing your thoughts vividly with enthusiasm favorably impresses everyone. Your large vocabulary, fluent speech, and clarity of thought causes a quiet authority to flow from you. Your powerful memory serves you well. Your manner of speaking inspires confidence in others and causes them to have a good opinion of you.

Each of these ideas is now making a permanent impression on your subconscious mind. Each day in your daily life you become more and more aware of the full and powerful expression of these ideas. Now, I am going to slowly count from one up to five. At the count of five, let your eyelids open. You're calm, rested, refreshed, relaxed, and you feel good. I'm going to give you a cassette recording that incorporates all the suggestions that you've just listened to and as you use it each day, you'll find that these ideas become a permanent part of your thinking, your feeling, your acting and reacting. Now that's just the way it will be. Not because I've said so, but because it's the nature of your mind to respond in this way.

As I count from one up to five, eyelids open, feeling

wonderfully good in every way. One, slowly, calmly, easily, and gently returning to your full awareness once again. Two, each muscle and nerve in your body is loose and limp and relaxed, and you feel good. Three, from head to toe you're feeling perfect in every way. On number four, you're beginning to feel sparkling clear. On the next number now, eyelids open, fully aware, feeling wonderfully good. Number five, eyelids open. Take a deep breath. Fill up your lungs and stretch. (Pat opens her eyes and has a big smile on her face.)

All right. You can pull your chair forward now. What was your thought and feeling about all that and those suggestions?

PAT: Well, as they were going past, I was imagining myself (Gil leans closer to Pat) doing them or agreeing with them.

BOYNE: Was there anything in there you couldn't agree with?

PAT: No, there was nothing that I couldn't agree with.

BOYNE: All of the suggestions were totally agreeable to you.

PAT: Right.

BOYNE: So each time you listen to them then, they'll become more and more a part of you.

PAT: (She nods affirmatively and smiles.) Thank you.

(Gil and Pat shake hands.)

BOYNE: Thank you.

What you've seen represents much of what we call hypnotism practice: that is, inducing a trance and programming powerful, creative, positive, and beneficial ideas which are specifically for the client. You notice that all the suggestions were positive. They all created mental imagery. They talked about what the client wanted. They didn't talk about the problem.

I spoke in the present tense because that's the only way the imagination can be truly excited in a positive way. It's this kind of programming that represents a large portion of hypnotism practice. Some of the other training films that you've seen utilize age regression and other uncovering techniques with certain kinds of problems, but in this situation we discovered there was no real phobia. There was no highly emotional- ized fear. There were no symptoms prior to each time Pat had to give a talk; there was no insomnia or vomiting, or any symptoms related to phobic per- formance anxiety. It becomes evident that simply reeducating the subconscious mind through creative reprogramming is the goal that we want to achieve.

I gave Pat an audio cassette titled "Secrets of Verbal Skills and Communication." The first side of the tape produces a trance using the "fractional relaxation" process, and it also utilizes suggestion programming so that a person responds easily and faster each time they go into trance. Once they acquire that skill, in just a few days, then they turn the tape over and listen to the programming that you just heard. This gives them a tool by which they continue to reinforce the ideas which symbolize the realization of their goal.

Until the next time, this is Gil Boyne.

HYPNOTHERAPY TO STOP PROJECTION OF CHILDHOOD FEARS

The Case of Holly ("You Scare Me")

A young woman in her mid-twenties breaks into tears in the first day of a clinical hypnotherapy course. When instructor Gil Boyne questions her, she says, "You're scaring me." This seems a paradox because Boyne has not spoken directly to her in class.

Boyne suggests that he hypnotize her to discover the background of her emotional upheaval. In minutes she is regressed to a terrifying scene with a threatening stepfather.

Abreaction, reeducation, rescripting, and closure each occur in rapid succession and the projected fear of an animated authority figure is dissipated.

THE CASE OF HOLLY
("You scare me")

BOYNE: Hello. This is Gil Boyne, and welcome again to the Hypnotherapy Video Clinic. Today we're here with Holly, who has an interesting story. Let's meet her now.

(BOYNE ADDRESS HOLLY)

HOLLY: Hi.

BOYNE: Holly, this is your second day in our Professional Hypnotism Training class, and a few moments ago we had a break and you came out teary-eyed and spoke to me about your feelings. Tell me about that now.

HOLLY: I told you that you scared me to death, the tone of your voice and sometimes the wording you use scared me. I mean, I am physically shaking now inside. (Holly's voice is quivering.)

BOYNE: When you say, "tone of voice and some of the words you use," give me an example of a word that scares you.

HOLLY: Probably swearing.

BOYNE: Such as.

HOLLY: I don't swear.

BOYNE: I didn't ask you if you swore. Give an idea of the word that I used.

HOLLY: You want me to say the word?

BOYNE: Yes.

HOLLY: You fucking so-and-so.

BOYNE: I never said that in class or out of class!

HOLLY: I thought I heard you say that.

BOYNE: I believe that you thought you heard me say it. Now I want you to be aware of what's going on in and around your eyes, your jaw, chest, and your stomach. Give a reporting starting with your eyes.

HOLLY: Wet.

BOYNE: You feel the moisture in your eyes. Now your chin and jaw.

HOLLY: Quivering.

BOYNE: Is what you're feeling in any way funny or humorous or entertaining to you?

HOLLY: No.

BOYNE: No, but you're smiling a lot.

HOLLY: Trying, yes.

BOYNE: Can you try to let the expression on your face match your feelings?

HOLLY: I don't know how to do that.

BOYNE: You see, when you smile, you're trying to discharge tensions and hold back your feelings at one and the same time.

HOLLY: Right.

BOYNE: And it's inappropriate because I know that what you're feeling is not appropriately displayed with a smile. Now you're here and it's okay for you to display your feelings. Go into your chest. What are you experiencing?

HOLLY: Tightness.

BOYNE: Tightness. Can you describe in a symbolic way, the tightness in your chest? "It feels like…" or "it feels as if…"

HOLLY: It's like there's a rock.

BOYNE: A rock in or on your chest.

HOLLY: Uh-huh.

BOYNE: And your stomach?

HOLLY: Kind of sick.

BOYNE: Describe the sickness. "It feels like, it feels as if..."

HOLLY: Like there's a lot of acid in it.

BOYNE: A churning in your stomach.

HOLLY: Uh-huh.

BOYNE: Now go into your head. What's the experience in your head?

HOLLY: Kind of lightheaded.

BOYNE: Put your hand on mine. Look at me. When I count to three, push down on my right hand. Keep looking at me. One, two, three. (Gil is using the Direct Gaze technique of induction) Begin pushing harder, harder, harder, eyelids heavy, droopy, drowsy, sleepy. They're closing, closing, closing, closing, closing, closing, closing, close them, close them, and SLEEP! (Gil places his hand on Holly's head and gently pushes her back in her reclining chair.) Now just turn loose, and let go. Let a good, pleasant feeling come all across your body. There's a feeling that has to do with being scared and feeling helpless, and as I count from one up to ten, you become very, very aware of that feeling. One, two, three, the feeling begins to emerge. Four, it's growing stronger now. It's a feeling of being frightened, scared. It's in the tone of the voice. It's the words. It's in the gestures, and you see them there. It's growing more and more intense, and you're feeling very small and very frightened and very upset.

Number five, six, seven, it's like the floodgates of a dam opening up now. Eight, it's rolling across you in a great wave. Nine, ten. (Gil places his hand on Holly's head and rotates it a bit.) This time I'll count to three and I'll tap your forehead. When I do, I'm going to ask you a question. The answer will come out by spelling, letter by letter. One, two, three. (Gil taps Holly's forehead.) Something causes you to feel fearful, frightened, and afraid. What is it now, the first letter?

HOLLY: V.

BOYNE: V, and the next.

HOLLY: O.

BOYNE: The next.

HOLLY: I.

BOYNE: The next.

HOLLY: C.

BOYNE: The next.

HOLLY: E.

BOYNE: VOICE. Now this time, I'll tap your forehead and a phrase, a sentence, or sentences will emerge using the word *voice*. (Gil taps Holly's head as he speaks the word) Now.

HOLLY: It's loud.

BOYNE: I'm going to count from ten down to one. As I do, we're going back to a time that has to do with this loud voice. Ten, nine, eight, you're drifting back. Seven, six, five, it has to do with this terrified feeling. Four, three, two, one. (Gil places his hand on Holly's head and shakes it a bit.) Where you are now, are you indoors or outside?

HOLLY: Indoors.

BOYNE: Is it daytime or nighttime?

HOLLY: Daytime.

BOYNE: You're indoors; it's in the daytime. Are you alone or is someone with you?

HOLLY: Someone's with me.

BOYNE: Who is it that's with you?

HOLLY: My dad.

BOYNE: How old are you?

HOLLY: Twelve.

BOYNE: You're twelve years old. Give a report on what's going on.

HOLLY: He's yelling at me.

BOYNE: I'll tap your forehead. Listen to what he's saying. (Gil taps Holly's forehead.)

HOLLY: He's calling me names.

BOYNE: Listen to the names. What is he calling you?

HOLLY: Son of a bitch. (Her voice is quivering.)

BOYNE: (Gil taps Holly's head.) Now listen to him again. What's he calling you?

HOLLY: The same thing.

BOYNE: Son of a bitch over and over, is that it?

HOLLY: Yes.

BOYNE: How do you feel as you see him behaving this way and calling you a "son of a bitch"?

HOLLY: Small.

BOYNE: Small. You're twelve years old. How old do you feel as you listen to him behave that way?

HOLLY: Two.

BOYNE: Two years old. All right. Do you love your father?

HOLLY: Yes.

BOYNE: Does he love you?

HOLLY: I think so.

BOYNE: Do you love your mother?

HOLLY: Yes.

BOYNE: Does she love you?

HOLLY: Yes.

BOYNE: Do you have any brothers or sisters?

HOLLY: Yes.

BOYNE: How many?

HOLLY: Two sisters.

BOYNE: Are they older or younger?

HOLLY: Older.

BOYNE: They're older. Do you ever get the feeling that your father loves or likes one of your sisters more than he likes you?

HOLLY: Yes.

BOYNE: Which one?

HOLLY: Both of them.

BOYNE: Both of them. Does he shout and call names to your sisters?

HOLLY: Not that I'm aware of.

BOYNE: Only to you; is that right?

HOLLY: Yes.

BOYNE: I'm going to count this time from seven down to one. We're going back to an earlier time that has to do with these very same feelings. Seven, six, five, growing younger now. Four, arms and legs are shrinking and you're growing smaller. Three, two, one. (Gil places his hand on Holly's head and shakes it a bit.) Are you indoors or outside?

HOLLY: Indoors.

BOYNE: Daytime or nighttime?

HOLLY: Nighttime.

BOYNE: Are you alone or is someone with you?

HOLLY: Someone is with me.

BOYNE: Who is it that's with you?

HOLLY: My dad.

BOYNE: How old are you?

HOLLY: Three.

BOYNE: You're three years old. You're with your dad. It's in the nighttime. Give a report on what's going on.

HOLLY: He's yelling at me.

BOYNE: He's yelling at you. What's he yelling? I'll tap your forehead. (Gil taps Holly's forehead.) Hear him yelling.

HOLLY: Telling me I can't do anything right.

BOYNE: You can't do anything right. You're only three years old. That's not a very good thing to say to a three-year-old, is it?

HOLLY: No.

BOYNE: What is it that you've done wrong?

HOLLY: Spilled something.

BOYNE: Spilled something. Well, every child that age spills a glass of milk or something once in awhile. How do you feel as you listen to him shout and holler?

HOLLY: Not too good.

BOYNE: Tell me the feeling in your body. What is it you're experiencing?

HOLLY: Sick.

BOYNE: Describe the sickness.

HOLLY: My stomach's upset.

BOYNE: Can you tell me "It feels like..." or "it feels as if..."?

HOLLY: I'm going to throw up.

BOYNE: Feels like you're going to throw up. Now in your chest.

HOLLY: It hurts.

BOYNE: It hurts. Describe it. "It feels like…"

HOLLY: A rock.

BOYNE: A rock is in your chest. Are you crying?

HOLLY: Yes.

BOYNE: All right. When I count to three, let your mind grow clear. One, two, three. (Gil places his hand on Holly's head as he says) Let your mind grow clear. Now you're three years old, and it's apparent that your father has a difficult time controlling his temper. I'm going to count from one up to seven. Come up to any age that you choose, that you feel is appropriate. I'm going to have you talk to your father. One, two, three, four, five, six, seven. (Gil is tapping Holly's head as he speaks to her.) All right. How old are you now?

HOLLY: Sixteen.

BOYNE: Sixteen. You're seated in the chair. Your father is seated out in the chair about eight feet in front of you. When I count to three (Gil taps Holly's forehead.), one, two three, there he sits. I want you to talk to him now. You're sixteen years old, and I want you to tell him, start out like this, say, "I want to tell you how I feel." What do you call him, Dad, Daddy?

HOLLY: Dad.

BOYNE: All right. Say, "Dad, I want to tell you how I feel."

HOLLY: Dad, I want to tell you how I feel.

BOYNE: Tell him. Now!

HOLLY: I feel hurt. I don't feel worth anything. I feel like I can't do anything right (tearful).

BOYNE: Tell him how you think that came about.

HOLLY: I think it's because you scare me. You make me feel that way. You yell at me all the time.

BOYNE: All right. Be the father. Your daughter says she feels worthless and she can't do anything right and it's your fault because of the way you yell at her all the time. Answer her.

HOLLY: (As the father) You know better than that. You know I love you, and I don't put you down, and you know that's not true.

BOYNE: Be the daughter. Your father says it's not true, and you should know better than that. Answer him.

HOLLY: It's because you yell at me and say those things.

BOYNE: Say to him, "When you yell at me, you scare me, and when you scare me, then I accept those ideas." Tell him that.

HOLLY: You yell at me and when you yell at me, you scare me, and I believe the things that you tell me when you yell at me.

BOYNE: All right, be the father. Answer your daughter.

HOLLY: (As the father) I don't mean to scare you.

BOYNE: Say it again.

HOLLY: I don't mean to scare you.

BOYNE: Say it again.

HOLLY: I don't mean to scare you.

BOYNE: I want you to tell your daughter how your father and your mother dealt with you in terms of hollering and scaring you. This is information you want to give her.

HOLLY: (As the father) My dad yelled at me all the time, but he didn't mean to scare me.

BOYNE: Tell your daughter if you ever felt frightened when your father yelled at you. Tell your daughter if you ever felt scared when you were a child and your father yelled at you.

HOLLY: (As the father) I used to be scared when my dad yelled at me.

BOYNE: Be the daughter. Answer that.

HOLLY: I get scared sometimes too.

BOYNE: Do you love your father?

HOLLY: Yes.

BOYNE: Can you tell him that?

HOLLY: Yes.

BOYNE: Tell him now.

HOLLY: I love you, Dad.

BOYNE: Can you ask him for something now or say, "I want to ask you to do something or not to do something"? Try it.

HOLLY: I want you to tell me you love me.

BOYNE: Be the father.

HOLLY: (As the father) I love you.

BOYNE: All right. Come back to yourself now. What's going on inside?

HOLLY: I feel kind of silly.

BOYNE: When I count from one up to ten, come up to this time and place. One, two, three, four, five, six, seven, eight, nine, ten. This is the month of June. It's 1985, June 11. I want you now when I count from three to do something different. I want you this time to use your adult, reasoning mind and to look back with that reasoning mind and examine the experiences of the child. See what she wanted from her father that she didn't get or what she got too much of; how it affected her and how those thoughts and feelings in those moments affected her behavior; how they affected her as she grew older; and how they are affecting you this very day. Take as much time as you need to figure it out. When you're ready to talk about it, just raise this arm up like this (Gil picks up Holly's right arm and demonstrates), and we'll talk about it.

All right, three, two, one. (Gil taps Holly's forehead as he counts down.) Now look back and analyze the experiences of the child. (Holly raises her right arm.) All right. Tell me about it. (Gil takes Holly's right hand as she begins to talk.)

HOLLY: I think she sometimes overexaggerated, but yet sometimes she wanted her father's attention so badly and then when she got it, it was negative. (Holly tries to hold back tears.)

BOYNE: Do you think that because she felt that Daddy loved the sisters more that she would rather have had the negative attention than no attention at all?

HOLLY: Could be.

BOYNE: And that maybe sometimes she produced or provoked the situation where he would holler? Did that ever occur?

HOLLY: Could be, but I don't think so.

BOYNE: You tell me how it was.

HOLLY: I think I tried to do everything I could to please my dad. He was too busy. He was very uncaring, didn't have time to say "I love you." Didn't have time to say, "You did a good job."

BOYNE: You know we all have a tendency to look back into our past and say, "I have had those feelings," or, "I feel unlovable," or, "I scared myself," and blame it on other people. "It's all because of what I didn't get from my parents." It seems like that is a very common tendency in people, but it's my belief that parents did what they did on the level of their own understanding. I have a feeling that you're still waiting for someone to behave in a different way so that you can feel validated. I have a feeling you're still out there trying to please everyone so they'll think you're nice and won't be angry at you. I have a feeling that you do a lot of placating. Is that true?

HOLLY: What's that mean?

BOYNE: *Placate* means to smooth things over.

HOLLY: Yeah.

BOYNE: Try to be nice, "I don't want any hard words" or—

HOLLY: That's true.

BOYNE: Paul said, "When I became a man, I put aside childish things," and I interpret that to mean that although it's true that as children we didn't have a way of defending ourselves against feelings of being unloved or feeling disapproved, as adults we must turn away from that constant focusing on what we didn't get. If some of our needs weren't filled, then it's up to us to find another way to fill them now. We're surrounded by people who have a capacity to love us, accept us, approve of us, and to nurture us, but until we become open to them, until we see the love and accept it, there is no healing that can take place. We starve in the midst of plenty because we're still looking back and saying, "Why didn't Dad love me more? Why wasn't he nicer to me?" We become a bottomless pit and the effort of others to love us does not nurture us and does not help us grow.

Now this time, I'm going to have you go back and sit there with your father, a little older now, and see if you can't bring a little more understanding to the situation, and a little more liberation, so that you can say good-by to your father and these psychic ties that bind you to him. All right. (Gil taps Holly's head as he counts) Three, two, one. There you sit in the chair, your father is out in front of you. How old are you this time?

HOLLY: Twenty.

BOYNE: Twenty years old. Now talk to your father. Say, "Dad, I want to tell you now about my real feelings."

HOLLY: Dad, I want to tell you how I feel. I feel like we need to be able to tell each other we love each other. I feel like we need to be honest with each other about how we feel. We need to be able to tell each other the things that have disappointed us about each other and talk about them and feel better about them.

BOYNE: Be the father. Answer your daughter.

HOLLY: (As the father) Sounds like a good idea to me.

BOYNE: Do you think now as you lie in your bed at night that you could continue this dialogue with your father and express these energies until you come to a closure?

HOLLY: Sure.

BOYNE: Go back into yourself. Be yourself. What's my name?

HOLLY: Gil.

BOYNE: The rest of it.

HOLLY: Boyne.

BOYNE: I'm Gil Boyne. How am I like your father?

HOLLY: Harsh.

BOYNE: How am I different from your father?

HOLLY: Your work's different, but you're a lot the same.

BOYNE: All right. Keep talking about the sameness.

HOLLY: Your looks, your hair, your tone of voice, your words, the way you talk, the way you act.

BOYNE: Now I have a question for you. Will you continue to scare yourself as you see some shadowy ghost when you look at me, or will you say, "Yes, he does express his energy in some of the same ways my father did, but his name is Gil Boyne, and he's not my father"? You have a choice of what you can do when you go back into that room. You can keep producing your funny little movies of the past and project them up on me and say, "Yes, there he is, just like my father." Or you can say, "No, he's harmless." Human beings do have certain characteristics in the way that they express their energy and there are a lot of similarities in many human beings.

HOLLY: Right.

BOYNE: Do you think you can handle that?

HOLLY: Yes.

BOYNE: All right. Now I'm going to ask the question a little differently. Very quickly now (Gil taps Holly's head.) Excluding your father, who else do I remind you of?

HOLLY: Gil Boyne.

BOYNE: Good. When I count from one up to five, let your eyelids open. You're calm, rested, refreshed, relaxed. You feel wonderfully good. One, slowly, calmly, easily, and gently returning to your full awareness once again. Two, each muscle and nerve in your body is loose and limp and relaxed. You feel good. Three, from head to toe, you're feeling perfect in every way. On number four, your eyes begin to feel sparkling clear. On the next number now, eyelids open, fully aware, feeling wonderfully good. Number five, eyelids open now. Take a deep breath. Fill up your lungs and stretch. (Holly is blowing her nose.) Well, you kind of surprised yourself, didn't you?

HOLLY: Yes.

BOYNE: Tell me about it.

HOLLY: Well, in a way I feel foolish. It seems like such a small thing to let control the inside of me. I feel like I can go finish the class now without sitting there on pins and needles and being afraid.

BOYNE: Get ready now. Are you ready?

HOLLY: I'm ready.

BOYNE: (Gil acts like a scary monster coming at Holly.) Boo!

HOLLY: I'm not scared of you, Gil Boyne! (Laughter. Gil and Holly shake hands.)

BOYNE: Congratulations.

HOLLY: Thank you.

(BOYNE ADDRESSES THE CAMERA)

BOYNE: Holly learned that when she said, "You're scaring me," it was really Holly scaring herself. It's easy to project an image of someone else onto an authority figure and then to say, "They're scaring me." That means, "They don't like me." Once you penetrate into the unreality of the childhood feelings of fear and then measure it against reality; you can put aside childish things. "As a child I saw through a glass darkly," said Paul. "As a man, I see clearly." Until the next time, this is Gil Boyne.

HYPNOTHERAPY TO CHANGE LIFESTYLES

The Case of Nancy ("You Make Me So Mad")

A young woman reports feelings of anger and rage towards Gil Boyne in the second day of hypnotherapy training. An intensive interview reveals the barrenness of her emotional life and her avoidance of social interactions.

Her use of her job (tour boat operator) as a control mechanism covers her cynicism, fear, and despair of having a meaningful relationship.

Age regression, "Parts" therapy, and Boyne's unique technique create a transformation which is immediately evident.

Three weeks later, Nancy begins training to acquire a real estate sales license. Eight months from the date of this session, she is working in realty sales full time. A transformation has occurred!

THE CASE OF NANCY
"You Make Me So Mad"

(BOYNE ADDRESSES THE AUDIENCE)

BOYNE: Hello. This is Gil Boyne. Welcome again to the Hypnotherapy Video Clinic. Today we're going to work with a class member. Let's meet her now.

(BOYNE ADDRESSES NANCY)

Tell me your name.

NANCY: Nancy.

BOYNE: Nancy, you began a week ago. You completed fifty hours of training in the first segment of the training program. This is the third day of our second course. Last night you asked to talk with me and expressed some feelings. Today you said you had a difficult time sleeping last night, and you've come to focus on some of these feelings, and you thought you wanted to work with them and see where it might lead you. Now tell me in your words what it is that's been bothering you.

NANCY: To start with, I feel that when you get excited or emotional about an issue, you get very loud, and that is very upsetting to me. I feel it's unnecessary, and I feel that it wastes class time.

BOYNE: When you spoke last night, you said you had spoken to one or two others who tend to agree with you. I want to point out that often when we feel an emotionalized response, we can turn to other people and state our feeling at the moment, and the easiest and best thing for them to do is to acknowledge some kind of an agreement. "Well, I can understand that. I can see how you feel that way, yes." Then to support our view, we can say, "See, they agree with me." But we don't want to deal with the other people now because none of them had trouble sleeping last night. You did.

NANCY: I don't know about that.

BOYNE: All right. They didn't report it to anyone else or to me. We want to deal with you and what I have viewed in you as I've looked at you in past the seven days. Many times you looked sad and most of the time when I spoke privately to you, there was a sullen appearance on your face, an angry, pouting look. I've seen this storm cloud around you a great deal of the time, and you're saying to me, "Well, every time you speak loudly or shout, I get angry."

NANCY: (She nods agreement.)

BOYNE: That anger is reflecting itself in your face and I'm seeing it.

NANCY: (She nods agreement.)

BOYNE: Since there are forty people in the room, let's say that there are two or three who agree with you, but the majority aren't upset. I think the key issue is that you said, "When I hear that loud shouting." You said, "My mind closes down and I can't learn."

NANCY: I get a headache. I don't listen, and what's going on in the room doesn't register with me.

BOYNE: So you leave the real environment—where you are— and you go somewhere else that you can't identify. Now let's move away from the classroom and see. Can you identify any other situations in which a similar response occurs?

NANCY: (She nods agreement.)

BOYNE: Tell me about those.

NANCY: I had a boss once who was very critical. And when he was critical about certain things, when he would say certain trigger things, I didn't listen to the rest of what he said. I didn't hear it. I—

BOYNE: Let me now interject. Initially you said "shouting," and now in this illustration it is "critical."

NANCY: (She nods agreement.) I have a similar feeling and a similar reaction.

BOYNE: They're almost interchangeable in producing your feelings—shouting produces a similar feeling to being criticized by an authority figure.

NANCY: (She nods agreement.)

BOYNE: So it may be that the two are linked together. Now, can you tell me of any memories of someone who shouted criticism at you?

NANCY: I don't remember anybody.

BOYNE: Tell me about your mother's temperament as you remember it.

NANCY: I used to call my mother the "Rock of Gibraltar." She had a very even, steady, strong temperament.

BOYNE: You emphasize the word *strong*. Tell me about that.

NANCY: She's a strong lady. I had an older sister who specialized in getting into trouble, and my mother managed not to let that create a lot of visible turmoil. I found out later that there was a lot of invisible turmoil, but with my mother it was, "That's not destroying my life and I'm not going to let that affect the way I treat my other children," so I used to call her the "Rock of Gibraltar."

BOYNE: Tell me about your father's emotional nature.

NANCY: My father's emotional nature. (Nancy smiles as she repeats these words.) Kind of a mystery to me. I don't know. I'm—I don't—I can't think of any words to describe it. He was not loud or silly.

BOYNE: Let me give you some choices and you can just say yes or no or maybe there's a place in between. Was your father aggressive or passive in his behavior?

NANCY: Towards me?

BOYNE: Was he an aggressive personality or a passive personality toward life?

NANCY: Towards business he's very aggressive.

BOYNE: In the family relationships?

NANCY: He was not aggressive. However, I wouldn't consider him passive either. He just got things done that needed to get done.

BOYNE: So he was effective.

NANCY: (She nods agreement.)

BOYNE: All right. You mention your mother as a "Rock of Gibraltar." Do you have kind of a similar characterization for your father? I don't mean the same one, but I mean a symbolic kind of description.

NANCY: No, my father is more of a mover. When something needed to get done, he sort of went ahead and did it.

BOYNE: He took action?

NANCY: Yes.

BOYNE: In that same category of taking action, what about your mother?

NANCY: She took action but not—again it wasn't visible. She said things that she thought would be effective, but she never struck out at us. She never forced us to do things, never forced us to go places.

BOYNE: Since you raised this issue, you said your feelings suddenly seem to overwhelm your thinking whenever someone is speaking in a loud manner. Were either of your parents prone to shouting?

NANCY: (She shakes her head negatively.) In fact, shouting was not allowed in our house.

BOYNE: Say that again.

NANCY: Shouting was not allowed in our house.

BOYNE: Once again.

NANCY: (Nancy chuckles as she says) Shouting was not allowed in our house.

BOYNE: All right. Can you remember anything that maybe your mother or father might have said as a communication about, "We don't allow shouting because..."

NANCY: There was never any because—it was just, "You're too loud," or "You're making too much noise," or my father's favorite line, "Quit your bellyaching." I remember hearing that most when my sisters and I would get in a scrape of some kind.

BOYNE: How do you think a child interpreted that statement, "Quit your bellyaching"? What meaning do you think was attached to it?

NANCY: Quit complaining or, you know, arguing.

BOYNE: Have you been married?

NANCY: No.

BOYNE: Never been married.

NANCY: (She shakes her head.)

BOYNE: How old are you now?

NANCY: Thirty-one.

BOYNE: Is your unmarried state a matter of personal choice— "I'm not interested in getting married," or "Not until I'm forty," or a matter of selection—"I've just never found the right one. I looked around, been engaged, but I decided this wasn't the right person for me," or some other reason?

NANCY: I'm not sure. I have always kept myself busy. (Nancy makes an indication of quote marks with her hands after the word *busy*.) Real busy, so there wasn't a great deal of space for someone—there wasn't a great deal of time for someone to get close to me, and I keep people at a distance.

BOYNE: You say, "I keep people at a distance." How would you characterize that in your relationships? What do you do to keep distance?

NANCY: I stay busy.

BOYNE: To me that sounds like, "I'm not available for dates, or to go off on a weekend," or whatever.

NANCY: (She nods agreement.)

BOYNE: Or am I saying it wrong? Maybe you're available for dates but not for relationships.

NANCY: Both of those things are true at different times. I went through a whole year period where I worked at least six days a week and usually seven, and they were ten-to-fifteen hour days.

BOYNE: What kind of work were you doing?

NANCY: I was working on a boat—charter boat.

BOYNE: Working in a vacation resort and having a constant flow of new people, it would seem like you had an opportunity to respond to requests for dates and so on. That kind of an atmosphere creates a lot of opportunity for good times.

NANCY: (She nods agreement.)

BOYNE: Did you have a great deal of opportunity for social activity all the time?

NANCY: A lot of the time I did and a lot of the time, I don't know, because again I kept myself so busy. I kept myself to one track on the boat totally. There wasn't any room for anybody to talk to me about anything else. I didn't allow it.

BOYNE: Say that again.

NANCY: I didn't allow anybody to talk to me about anything but business.

BOYNE: Right, but I can imagine someone running the boat and still being social, getting invitations.

NANCY: Uh-huh.

BOYNE: But if you don't allow anyone to talk to you about anything other than business then you're controlling them.

NANCY: (She nods agreement.) I didn't like most of the people I saw that were running boats and spending a lot of time partying. I didn't like them at all.

BOYNE: Do you think there is a middle ground—other than working all the time and not allowing anyone to talk about social activities and making partying a central theme of one's existence?

NANCY: I hope so. I haven't found it yet. (Laughter from both Gil and Nancy.)

BOYNE: You have never occupied the middle ground yet.

NANCY: Right.

BOYNE: All right. Close your eyes, please. I'm going to give you the beginning of a sentence, and I want you to repeat it and finish it. "So long as I stay busy, I..."

NANCY: So long as I stay busy, people won't know that I am lonely.

BOYNE: Very good. Start again and put a new ending on it.

NANCY: So long as I stay busy, people can't hurt my feelings.

BOYNE: Once again put a new ending on it.

NANCY: So long as I stay busy, I don't have to think about what I'm going to do the rest of my life.

BOYNE: Try again.

NANCY: So long as I stay busy, I don't have to do a lot of little things—laundry and dishes. I can avoid those things.

BOYNE: Does that mean, "I work more to make more money and then pay someone else to do my laundry and dishes"?

NANCY: Hopefully—I never got to that point.

BOYNE: (Chuckle) All right.

NANCY: (Chuckle) That's what I was hoping for.

BOYNE: Sounds like your life has been kind of one-sided, or unbalanced is a better word. What have you done for play or fun or filling some of those needs for relationship?

NANCY: What do you mean?

BOYNE: If you didn't party and you didn't let people on the boat talk to you and ask you for dates because you're too busy, what did you do? Did you develop a hobby? Did you say, "I'll just listen to classical music three hours a day"? Did you write a journal? What did you do?

NANCY: I did a lot of extra work on the boat. I took a project of training some of the girls who were tired of not being able to move up in their position. I did do a lot of partying with a lot of people, and it wasn't for me.

BOYNE: Let's talk about that. "It wasn't for me because..."

NANCY: In Lahaina mostly it wasn't for me because of the drugs and the drinking and the craziness.

BOYNE: You felt that you weren't in the same place they were; you didn't feel the need for the use of alcohol and other drugs and behavior that you felt just didn't suit you or wasn't very good for you.

NANCY: I felt it was harmful.

BOYNE: All right.

NANCY: I mean, I tried a lot of those things and some of them lasted longer than others and some of them didn't work out. Some of them did more damage to me than others. Long before anybody else, I thought, "This is only hurting me," and stopped.

BOYNE: Now you're indicating that you were a drug user at one time.

NANCY: Right.

BOYNE: And you became aware of the harmful effects.

NANCY: (She nods agreement.)

BOYNE: What were the harmful effects that you discovered for yourself, the effects that caused you to change your mind?

NANCY: Well, the biggest, the most memorable one was at one point when I was living with some people. There were four of us who lived in a house, and all we did was take drugs and play cards and watch TV and take drugs and play cards and watch TV. And after a couple of months, I noticed the people around me getting paranoid. I noticed one of them starting to carry a gun and that scared me, and more and more people were coming to the back door wanting drugs. And I was like, "Wait a minute, everybody is beginning to know that this is going on here and pretty soon the police are going to know," and then I started getting paranoid. When I got paranoid, I started becoming aware of the other effects, and like I wasn't breathing properly or I could only—I used to do yoga and there's some stretches I could only do when I was high and that didn't make sense. It was like, well, if my mind was controlling it, then I should be able to do it without the drugs but couldn't. And so there was like a grip there.

BOYNE: I hear you saying you felt you were losing control or out of control.

NANCY: (She nods agreement.)

BOYNE: Which one fits?

NANCY: I was losing control.

BOYNE: So you then regained your control by discontinuing that kind of behavior.

NANCY: Yes, I moved out of the house.

BOYNE: All right. So far it seems to me that you said you've gone from one place to the other—from devoting a lot of your energy to pleasure to total devotion to work.

NANCY: I always work with pleasure. (Nancy smiles as she says this.)

BOYNE: The pleasure of...

NANCY: Being on the ocean and being with people. I always have new people on the boat every day.

BOYNE: What's the benefit of always being with new people?

NANCY: I got to hear a lot of different things from a lot of different places around the world. I got a lot of different opinions and viewpoints, and I learned a lot from those people, and I didn't have to change my routine. (Laughter from both Gil and Nancy.)

BOYNE: Say that again.

NANCY: I could tell them the same jokes day after day and always had a new audience to laugh.

BOYNE: You didn't have to worry that they might come to know you too well or see inside you too far—

NANCY: (She nods agreement.)

BOYNE: —and maybe get a glimpse of you as you believed you were inside.

NANCY: (She nods agreement.)

BOYNE: That's called superficial relationships, whether it's characterized in the way you were doing it or the gal who goes down to the singles bar every night and brings home a different guy to help her make it through the night. That's a contact without involvement. Avoidance of intimacy, is that what we're talking about?

NANCY: Probably.

BOYNE: Push your chair back. Put your hand in mine. When I count to three, press down as hard as you can. One, look at me. Two, pressing down harder. Press it down harder. All the force you can muster now—even harder, harder. Eyelids heavy, droopy, drowsy, sleepy. Close them and sleep. (Gil releases his hand from Nancy's as he says the word *sleep*.) That's good. Now just let every muscle and nerve (Gil shakes Nancy's hand limply from side to side as he says this) just grow loose and limp and relaxed. There's a feeling that you are aware of. It's a feeling of someone shouting loudly, and as you begin to picture that—their arms waving and their voices so loud—you begin to feel angry. You begin to feel great rage boiling up. Now your mind is becoming a blank.

As I count from one up to ten, I want you to become aware of that feeling. One, two, three, the feeling is growing stronger and stronger now. Four, it's rolling across you in a great wave. Five, a great, powerful, intense wave rolling across you now. Six, it's like the floodgates on a dam opening up. Seven, the shouting is loud, angry, and you're feeling more and more angry. Your mind is just closing down now. Nine, it seems like it's more intense than you ever felt it before. Number ten. I'm going to count to three. I'll ask you a question. The answer will come out by spelling letter by letter. One, two, three. (Gil taps Nancy's forehead as he asks) What is it that causes you to have these feelings? The first letter. Quickly, the first letter.

NANCY: "P"

BOYNE: The next. Quickly, the next letter.

NANCY: It's a preacher.

BOYNE: A preacher. When I touch your forehead, I want you to make a sentence or a phrase that has to do with the preacher. (Gil taps Nancy's forehead.)

NANCY: He's screaming.

BOYNE: I'm going to count from ten down to one. As I do, we'll go back to an earlier time that has to do with these feelings. Ten, nine, eight, you're drifting back. Seven, six, five, growing younger now. Four, your arms and legs are shrinking. You're growing smaller. Three, two, one. (Gil taps Nancy's head.) Where you are now, are you indoors or outside? Make a choice. Pick one.

NANCY: It's blank.

BOYNE: I asked are you indoors or outside. Pick one.

NANCY: I'm indoors.

BOYNE: Daytime or nighttime?

NANCY: Nighttime.

BOYNE: You're indoors and it's nighttime. Are you alone or is someone with you?

NANCY: I'm alone.

BOYNE: How do you feel?

NANCY: Quiet.

BOYNE: "I feel quiet." How old are you?

NANCY: I don't know.

BOYNE: I didn't say choose from "yes, no, or I don't know." Are you younger than fourteen years old, yes or no?

NANCY: Yes.

BOYNE: Are you younger than twelve years old, yes or no?

NANCY: Yes.

BOYNE: Are you younger than ten years old, yes or no?

NANCY: Yes.

BOYNE: Are you younger than eight years old, yes or no?

NANCY: Yes.

BOYNE: Are you younger than six years old, yes or no?

NANCY: No.

BOYNE: Are you six years old?

NANCY: No.

BOYNE: Are you seven years old, yes or no?

NANCY: Yes.

BOYNE: All right. You're seven years old. Now you're seven years old. It's nighttime and you're indoors and you feel "quiet." What's happening to your voice as you report feeling quiet?

NANCY: It's very quiet.

BOYNE: Your voice is very quiet. How do you feel about that quiet feeling?

NANCY: It's all right.

BOYNE: Is that something that you experience often?

NANCY: No.

BOYNE: You're seven years old. Are you in your house now?

NANCY: (She nods agreement.)

BOYNE: Where is your mother?

NANCY: I don't know.

BOYNE: Do you love your mother?

NANCY: Yes.

BOYNE: Does she love you?

NANCY: Yes.

BOYNE: Where's your father?

NANCY: I don't know.

BOYNE: Do you love your father?

NANCY: (She nods agreement.)

BOYNE: Does he love you?

NANCY: (She nods agreement.) Yes.

BOYNE: You had a smile as you said that. (Nancy chuckles.) Tell me about the smile.

NANCY: He used to play with us. He used to take us water skiing, and I was too young to water ski.

BOYNE: You were too small to water ski but you remember the good times and the pleasures with the children.

NANCY: (She nods agreement.)

BOYNE: All right. Do you have brothers and sisters?

NANCY: I have two sisters.

BOYNE: You're seven. How old are your sisters?

NANCY: Eleven, thirteen.

BOYNE: Eleven and thirteen. Do you love your sisters?

NANCY: Yeah.

BOYNE: Do they love you?

NANCY: Yeah.

BOYNE: Is there anything that goes on in the family that's upsetting to you?

NANCY: I can't water ski. I don't want to learn.

BOYNE: Say it again.

NANCY: I don't want to learn to water ski. I'm afraid of the— but I want to water ski.

BOYNE: You want to do it so you can be like the other kids, but you're afraid of doing it, is that right?

NANCY: (She nods agreement.)

BOYNE: When I tap your forehead, you can complete a sentence. (Gil taps Nancy's forehead.) Say, "I'm afraid if I were on the water skis..."

NANCY: I might fall down.

BOYNE: I'm going to count from four down to one. As I do, we're going back to a time that has to do with that feeling of falling down. Four, three, two, one. (Gil places his hand on Nancy's head and says) Are you indoors or outside? Quickly.

NANCY: I'm outside.

BOYNE: Daytime or nighttime?

NANCY: Daytime.

BOYNE: Are you alone or is someone with you?

NANCY: There is somebody with me.

BOYNE: Who is it that's with you?

NANCY: The twins.

BOYNE: The twins. How old are they? How old are you?

NANCY: I don't know.

BOYNE: Are you younger than seven years old?

NANCY: (She nods agreement.)

BOYNE: Are you younger than six years old?

NANCY: (She nods agreement.)

BOYNE: Are you younger than five years old? Are you five years old?

NANCY: Maybe.

BOYNE: All right. You're with the twins. You're outside. What's going on? Give a report.

NANCY: Running through the sprinklers.

BOYNE: "Running through the sprinklers." I bet that feels good.

NANCY: (She nods agreement.)

BOYNE: Having fun?

NANCY: (She nods agreement.)

BOYNE: You're running through the sprinklers. Who's with you?

NANCY: The twins.

BOYNE: "The twins." Are the twins from your family?

NANCY: (She shakes her head negatively and puts her right hand over her eyes.)

BOYNE: How do you feel?

NANCY: Dizzy.

BOYNE: "I feel dizzy." Can you describe the dizziness?

NANCY: Just the world looks crooked.

BOYNE: All right. Just keep coming forward minute by minute. What's happening?

NANCY: The twins' mother is watching us. It seems like there are a lot of kids running through the sprinklers, and I'm just standing and watching them.

BOYNE: What is happening with the dizziness?

NANCY: I just feel dizzy.

BOYNE: What do you feel in your body?

NANCY: Kind of like—like I'm standing on something that isn't straight. I almost feel like I want to fall over but I'm not falling.

BOYNE: Is that feeling linked to the dizziness? "I feel dizzy and like I want to fall over."

NANCY: Yes.

BOYNE: Have you ever had this dizziness before in this way?

NANCY: (Long pause) No.

BOYNE: And now?

NANCY: I'm just standing there.

BOYNE: What is it that keeps you separated from the other kids and not joining in to have such a good time running through the sprinklers?

NANCY: I don't know.

BOYNE: Do you like any of those kids—the twins and so on?

NANCY: (She nods affirmatively.)

BOYNE: Do they like you?

NANCY: Yes.

BOYNE: Do you ordinarily like to play with them?

NANCY: (She nods agreement.)

BOYNE: What's happening today?

NANCY: I don't know.

BOYNE: You made a sound with your mouth (as if Nancy is blowing air from her mouth). Do that again. Again.

NANCY: (The sound is made by Nancy.)

BOYNE: Once again. As you do, let it fill up—form in your mind.

NANCY: (She makes the sound again.)

BOYNE: How is the day different?

NANCY: There's something glaring in my eye.

BOYNE: You mean like the sun or reflection—a person?

NANCY: There's a light right in front of me.

BOYNE: Where is that light coming from?

NANCY: (Nancy is pointing as she says) Up there.

BOYNE: You think it's looking at the light that makes you dizzy?

NANCY: I don't know.

BOYNE: All right. Let your mind grow clear. And I'll count up to four and we're going back to another time and place when you're seven years old. One, two, three, four. (Gil places his hand on Nancy's head for a moment.) Now you are back at seven. How do you feel?

NANCY: Fine.

BOYNE: What's going on? Give a report.

NANCY: (Nancy smiles as she says) We're taking popcorn off the cobs.

BOYNE: Popping corn—taking it off the cobs.

NANCY: Uh-huh.

BOYNE: Is that fun?

NANCY: Uh-huh.

BOYNE: You like doing that?

NANCY: Uh-huh.

BOYNE: Who are you doing it with?

NANCY: The whole neighborhood.

BOYNE: "The whole neighborhood." Is this corn that everybody grew?

NANCY: No.

BOYNE: "No." Corn you bought?

NANCY: No.

BOYNE: Where did the corn come from?

NANCY: My uncle sent it to me.

BOYNE: I see. It was a gift to you and you're sharing it with the neighborhood.

NANCY: (She nods agreement.)

BOYNE: Wonderful. Do you have a lot of friends?

NANCY: Yeah.

BOYNE: Do you like to play with your friends and be with them?

NANCY: (She nods agreement.)

BOYNE: Do your friends like you?

NANCY: (She nods agreement.)

BOYNE: I'll count from one up to four, we'll go up to a time and place where you're older. One, two, three, four. (Gil taps Nancy's forehead and says) Where you are now, are you indoors or outside?

NANCY: I'm outside.

BOYNE: Daytime or nighttime?

NANCY: Nighttime.

BOYNE: Are you alone or is someone with you?

NANCY: Someone's with me.

BOYNE: Who is it that's with you?

NANCY: The school kids.

BOYNE: How old are you?

NANCY: I think I'm eight.

BOYNE: Eight years old. What's going on?

NANCY: They're taunting me.

BOYNE: Taunting you. What are they taunting you about?

NANCY: (Nancy smiles and says) I'm a new kid in school.

BOYNE: I see. You just moved into that area?

NANCY: Yes.

BOYNE: When I touch your forehead, you'll become aware of

some things some of these kids are saying as taunts. (Gil taps Nancy's forehead.) What is it they're saying?

NANCY: That I lied to them; that I'm not really from California.

BOYNE: Did you lie?

NANCY: No.

BOYNE: "No." All right. How do you feel that they call you a liar?

NANCY: I'm upset.

BOYNE: Is anyone shouting it at you?

NANCY: (She nods agreement.)

BOYNE: Yeah.

NANCY: (Nancy sighs deeply.)

BOYNE: Is there anyone like the boys jumping up and down waving their arms?

NANCY: (She nods negatively.)

BOYNE: Just hollering at you?

NANCY: All the girls.

BOYNE: "All the girls." Are they making any kind of movements as they holler?

NANCY: (Tears are running down Nancy's face.) No.

BOYNE: "No." When I tap your forehead, hear one more girl saying something. (Gil taps Nancy's forehead as he says) What is it you hear?

NANCY: Something about money.

BOYNE: All right. Listen again. Hear it more clearly. (Gil taps Nancy's forehead.) Be the money. Listen now.

NANCY: That I must be spoiled and I must be a brat because my father has money.

BOYNE: I see. How do you feel about that?

NANCY: I don't know what they mean. (Nancy is crying as she says this.)

BOYNE: No, I don't either.

NANCY: I don't know what it means. (Nancy is crying hard at this point.)

BOYNE: When I count to three, let your mind grow clear. (Gil places his hand on Nancy's head.) One, two, three. Just let it grow clear now, clear and calm. I'm going to count from one up to ten. Come up to this time and place. One, two, three, four, five, six, seven, eight, nine, ten. This is the month of August. It is 1985, and you're a grown woman now.

I'm going to count from three to one. I want you to look back at this child and those experiences and see what kind of thoughts and feelings developed in her and how those thoughts and feelings affected her behavior as she grew and how they're affecting you even this very moment as you sit in this training class. Look back and analyze, and when you're ready to talk about it, bring your hand up (Gil takes Nancy's left hand and demonstrates what he wants) on your chest and we'll talk further about it now. (Gil taps Nancy's forehead as he says) Three, two, one. Now look back and analyze the experiences of this child. (Long pause.) Are you ready to talk about it?

NANCY: I guess so.

BOYNE: (Gil holds Nancy's hand as he says) What happened to the child and how does she think and feel?

NANCY: I didn't understand. I didn't know why they hated me. I didn't know what money had to do with it. I didn't know what money was.

BOYNE: What do you think is the message the child got from those other kids?

NANCY: If you're different, people hate you.

BOYNE: "If you're different, people hate you." How about, if you have money or the family has money? Start with that sentence.

NANCY: If your family has money, people envy you.

BOYNE: Good.

NANCY: People don't know what they're talking about.

BOYNE: I want you to just imagine for a moment you're back being that child and make this statement as the child. "When I grow up..." and then tell me what you're going to do or how it's going to be that will make a difference.

NANCY: When I grow up nobody is ever going to make me feel this way again.

BOYNE: That's very good. Start again and put a new ending on it.

NANCY: When I grow up, I'm never going to listen to them.

BOYNE: Very good. Start again. Put a new ending on it.

NANCY: (Nancy is sighing deeply during this time) I'm never going to hate anybody for having money.

BOYNE: "I'm never going to hate anyone for having money." Start again. Say, "When I grow up..."

NANCY: When I grow up, I'm never going to get in a bunch of girls again.

BOYNE: That's very good. Now one more time. Say, "When I grow up..." and put an ending on it.

NANCY: When I grow up, I'm never going to have money.

BOYNE: (Gil places his hand on Nancy's forehead and says) Come back to this time and place now. And this time when I tap your forehead, we're going to say something and do something that has to do with this feeling of anger when someone's shouting or waving their arm. (Gil taps Nancy's forehead.) All right. Now connect if you can with the feeling of anger that you get that keeps you from thinking and learning.

NANCY: I don't know what they're talking about.

BOYNE: And that makes you feel angry, frustrated.

NANCY: Yes.

BOYNE: Can you see how certain situations cause you to get stuck at that place in your feelings—that place where you felt it was so unfair and so unjust?

NANCY: Yes.

BOYNE: You can see how the child got to feel that way, can't you, because it really was unfair. It was really unjust. On the other hand, it was the cruel kind of behavior that kids indulge in at certain ages.

NANCY: They still do.

BOYNE: "They still do." Kids still do or adults still behave toward you that way?

NANCY: People still behave towards me that way.

BOYNE: Which is?

NANCY: Unfair.

BOYNE: So, "I'm always being treated unfairly."

NANCY: I'm very often being treated unfairly.

BOYNE: Give me an example.

NANCY: People think they know what I'm all about and they don't.

BOYNE: "People make judgments of me on superficial experience of me"?

NANCY: Yes.

BOYNE: "And that makes me feel..."

NANCY: I get angry. I don't want to be like them. I don't want to be around them.

BOYNE: Okay. Now, "People make judgments of me on limited or superficial knowledge of me." How does that relate to me?

NANCY: They're wrong.

BOYNE: How does that relate to me, Gil Boyne?

NANCY: I don't know.

BOYNE: Are you aware that last week especially I demonstrated how just through a few sentences or even a few words a person might speak that one could begin to process certain ideas about them, and I illustrated it with several people in the room when they spoke?

NANCY: I don't know what you mean.

BOYNE: People would make a certain statement, and I would say it sounds like beneath that statement such and such—

NANCY: (She has her right arm over her mouth as Gil speaks.)

BOYNE: —and go down maybe six or eight or ten different statements, and they would say, "Yes, that's right." Then I would say, "If you would listen to what the people are saying, you can pick up a lot in just a few sentences." You just said you feel it's unfair for people to draw conclusions based on a little bit of knowledge or information. Do you relate that feeling of anger, unfairness to that same thing that I do as part of a clinical practice?

NANCY: No.

BOYNE: All right. Is there anything that you can come up with now that says to you, "When that man raises his voice and waves his arms, I get very upset," anything that connects with it as a result of your memories and your feelings being open right now?

NANCY: You—you seem to put things down without thinking about them.

BOYNE: Just like—

NANCY: Just like those girls put me down without knowing who I was.

BOYNE: And that's unfair.

NANCY: Yes.

BOYNE: "So every time you seem angry and critical, Gil Boyne, you trigger me back to that scene with the girls in my feelings."

NANCY: Yes.

BOYNE: What are we going to do about that?

NANCY: Forget it.

BOYNE: Well, you don't really ever forget anything. Hopefully now that you're more aware of it, you won't react or you'll check your reaction. You have great power. You checked your flight into drugs. You checked your flight into inappropriate behavior and you governed it and controlled it and now that you have a greater understanding, I'm sure you'll check this feeling when it's not really someone directing energy toward you. Can you agree to start working on that?

NANCY: (Nancy's eyes are moist.) Yes.

BOYNE: Fine. Is there anything more that you would like to say to me, ask me, or tell me in this session?

NANCY: With all the power, I'm out of control.

BOYNE: "I feel out of control."

NANCY: I just feel out of control.

BOYNE: Here's a beginning: "If I ever really let go..." or "If I ever really let loose..." Put an ending on it.

NANCY: If I ever really let loose, I'd be crazy.

BOYNE: Start again and put a new ending on it.

NANCY: If I ever really let loose, I won't be able to do anything.

BOYNE: "I'd be..." what—paralyzed, immobilized?

NANCY: (She nods agreement.)

BOYNE: One more time. "If I ever really..."

NANCY: If I ever really let go, I might kill myself.

BOYNE: So you really do struggle for control a lot of the time, don't you. And so if it appears to you that I am out of control, then that's very frightening, isn't it?

NANCY: (She nods agreement.)

BOYNE: "Good lord, there's someone out of control and I'll be next." All right. In a moment I'm going to get you up. You're going to realize the great power and strength within you and your ability to direct it in your own behalf. You're going to feel like a great weight has come off your chest or off your shoulders or off your stomach. Very quickly now, who do I remind you of?

NANCY: Baptist preacher.

BOYNE: How am I like the Baptist preacher?

NANCY: You scream a lot.

BOYNE: What qualities other than screaming do I share with a Baptist minister?

NANCY: You have white hair.

BOYNE: White hair. One more thing.

NANCY: The other day you wore a very dark shirt and a dark suit with a white collar, and you just looked like a Baptist minister.

BOYNE: All right. Well, I'm neither Baptist nor a minister. I hope you'll reassure yourself of that no matter what my behavior is. Is that agreeable to you?

NANCY: I don't know.

BOYNE: You will think it over? You're going to have a much better sleep tonight than you had last night. That's agreeable, isn't it?

NANCY: (She nods agreement.)

BOYNE: You'll have a wonderful night's sleep tonight, one of the best night's sleep of your entire life. When I count from one to five, let your eyelids open. You're calm, rested, refreshed, relaxed. You feel good. One, slowly, calmly, easily, and gently returning to your full awareness once again. Two, each muscle and nerve in your body is loose and limp and relaxed. You feel good. Three, from head to toe you're feeling perfect in every way. On number four, your eyes begin to feel sparkling clear. On the next number now, eyelids open, fully aware, feeling wonderfully good. Number five, eyelids open now. Take a deep breath. Fill up your lungs and stretch. Bring your chair up. We've got just a few minutes left. What do you think of all that?

NANCY: I still don't know what hypnotism is.

BOYNE: (Gil taps Nancy's hand and says) What do you think about the feelings you felt and what you had to say? What's your initial reaction to it now?

NANCY: I'm surprised that I remembered those girls today. I remembered them a lot of other times in my life. I'm surprised that I remembered them today.

BOYNE: We call that an "initial sensitizing event." There was a powerful pool of energy that became sensitized and locked in right at that point, and you keep going back to it a lot, don't you?

NANCY: (She nods agreement.)

           (BOYNE ADDRESSES CAMERA)

BOYNE: The "initial sensitizing event" is often just that. It's a place where a feeling develops. It becomes a pool of energy and as various experiences occur in life, a tentacle seems to form a connection between the experience and this pool of energy. Soon more and more tentacles emerge until this original pool of energy can have many, many connections to many different kinds of situations. The only way we can change the nature or quality of the pool of energy is to change the underlying ideas, the fixed ideas that were part of the "initial sensitizing event," then the tentacles weaken and wither. Beyond that there are many secondary reinforcing events. Each time one of these experiences triggers the old emotional playback and the same reaction occurs, it is a reinforcement that makes us feel more certain about our perception even though it is distorted by a cloud of unreality brought upon us by our emotions.

Until the next time, this is Gil Boyne.

HYPNOTHERAPY TO FIND LOST OBJECTS

The Case of Claudia ("The Lost Diamond Necklace")

A young married woman has lost or mislaid an expensive diamond necklace and cannot remember her handling of it. Her comic style and low self-esteem create difficulties in the hypnotic session.

In a sudden, unexpected conclusion, Boyne pushes Claudia through her memory block and she "remembers" where she hid the necklace.

THE CASE OF CLAUDIA
"The Lost Diamond Necklace"

(BOYNE ADDRESSES THE AUDIENCE)

BOYNE: Hello. This is Gil Boyne, and welcome to another session of the Hypnotherapy Video Clinic. Today we're with Claudia, and this is our first meeting.

(BOYNE ADDRESSES CLAUDIA)

Hello.

CLAUDIA: Ciao.

BOYNE: How can I help you today, Claudia?

CLAUDIA: Gosh, I hope so. I lost a diamond. I hid it. I — let's see. The last time I saw it was in my husband's office in some files; and I took it, but I don't know what I did with it after that. It was in a little thing.

BOYNE: A little box?

CLAUDIA: Yeah, a little box with some costume jewelry.

BOYNE: Was this diamond a ring, an earring?

CLAUDIA: A necklace.

BOYNE: A necklace.

CLAUDIA: It was about three carats I think. I don't have a clue what it would be worth. It had a slight—it was cloudy. It was rather nice, and then I wanted to wear it one day and I couldn't find it.

BOYNE: Well, let's say it's expensive to say the least.

CLAUDIA: Yeah, I—I don't know, $5,000 maybe.

BOYNE: How long ago was it that you lost or misplaced the diamond?

CLAUDIA: About two months. I got married March 28.

BOYNE: Nineteen eighty five.

CLAUDIA: (She nods in agreement.)

BOYNE: Was there anything associated with your seeing this diamond—was it a discovery, a surprise, a treat? Did it make you curious or was it just that you knew it was there and you went to look at it and that's how it came about?

CLAUDIA: Oh, how I discovered I misplaced it?

BOYNE: No. Let's start with the actual discovery of the diamond. Did you know the diamond was in that box?

CLAUDIA: Uh-huh.

BOYNE: So it wasn't a surprise, wasn't anything that had been hidden from you?

CLAUDIA: No.

BOYNE: Or a surprise gift to you or anything that affected you emotionally?

CLAUDIA: It was—Oh, maybe, yeah.

BOYNE: Tell me about it.

CLAUDIA: Well, I hid it because since we were going to get married and I was scared, someone might find it in my apartment, so—

BOYNE: While you were on your honeymoon?

CLAUDIA: Right. So I hid it in his office, and he wanted to put it in his safety deposit box.

BOYNE: I see.

CLAUDIA: And I decided no, no, I'll hide it amongst these files. (Claudia chuckles. She reminds you of Goldie Hawn in her looks and her attitude.) I guess that's it. Before that an old boyfriend gave it to me. So maybe that's how come. I was supposed to marry him, and I cancelled the wedding three days before, so maybe that's why I misplaced it, because I really didn't want to find it.

BOYNE: So you think, "Maybe there's an emotional connection in that it is a gift from a former lover who wanted to marry me and just three days before the wedding I broke it off."

CLAUDIA: (Laughter.)

BOYNE: "And this reminds me of him."

CLAUDIA: Yeah, maybe, yeah.

BOYNE: Is that a possibility?

CLAUDIA: Yeah.

BOYNE: We may never know, but it is a possibility.

CLAUDIA: Yeah, yeah, and—never mind. There's more, but I don't want to go into it.

BOYNE: How long has it been—March? Did you say March 20?

CLAUDIA: Twenty-eighth.

BOYNE: Twenty-eighth. April, May, little over two months.

CLAUDIA: (She nods in agreement.) It could have been pinched, you never know.

BOYNE: You took it out and that's the last memory you have of it?

CLAUDIA: Well, okay. Okay. January, February, March, so it was a week after that. I took it and I was cleaning out my flat because I was moving, and I don't know what I did with it from there. I could have left it in my car. I could have left it anywhere.

BOYNE: Or it could have been found by someone else?

CLAUDIA: Precisely. That's what I was saying, you know.

BOYNE: All right.

CLAUDIA: Expensive mistake. (She giggles.)

BOYNE: What led you here?

CLAUDIA: My husband actually. A friend of his, David Wright. You might know David. He knew of you. He sold you a house or something, and he said you were a great hypnotist.

BOYNE: I own several properties, but I don't—

CLAUDIA: Yeah, I think—he's a real estate agent, anyway. He took care of it all. He made the appointment and here I am.

BOYNE: Now that you're here, how do you feel about it so far?

CLAUDIA: I've never been hypnotized before. So, I don't know. Maybe you can't even hypnotize me. Well, you never know, right? (Laughs)

BOYNE: Actually hypnosis is a natural state of mind, which means everyone has a natural capacity for response. Some respond a little easier than others, but everyone can respond.

CLAUDIA: Oh, really? Oh, okay. (She is giggling.)

BOYNE: Have you ever seen anyone hypnotized?

CLAUDIA: Yeah, once, a long time ago.

BOYNE: Tell me about that.

CLAUDIA: Actually, I forget where.

BOYNE: Nightclub?

CLAUDIA: Something like that.

BOYNE: Do you remember any thoughts or feelings you had about it?

CLAUDIA: No, I can't recall, I guess. I'm just really frightened actually.

BOYNE: Did you get to talk to any of the people after they came off the stage?

CLAUDIA: No, it was really crowded, and we were in the back.

(She has her head down and appears very nervous.)

BOYNE: Many people seeing that kind of a show think that hypnosis is a kind of state in which you'll do anything that is suggested, that you behave compulsively and you have no controls. But you have to think about it. What kind of people went on the stage to volunteer?

CLAUDIA: I guess kind of extroverts.

BOYNE: Yes. Or even exhibitionists or people who at least were willing to perform in front of a group.

CLAUDIA: Yeah.

BOYNE: You didn't volunteer, did you?

CLAUDIA: Oh, no, no, never. (She shakes her head back and forth as she says this and laughs.)

BOYNE: So you exercised your control by not going up on the stage.

CLAUDIA: Uh-huh.

BOYNE: They exercised their control by going up, didn't they?

CLAUDIA: (She nods in agreement.)

BOYNE: Then they did things that they had agreed to do in advance before they came up on the stage.

CLAUDIA: Oh, I see.

BOYNE: They said, "I'm going up and have fun."

CLAUDIA: (She laughs a little and says) Yeah, I guess. You had to have two drinks or something, you know, so maybe they were hoping, I don't know.

BOYNE: But in hypnotism you do have measures of control and there's no way that you can accept suggestions that are against your values or character attitudes or religious beliefs. There never has been such a case in history.

CLAUDIA: Oh, really?

BOYNE: (He nods affirmatively.)

CLAUDIA: Oh.

BOYNE: That surprises you, doesn't it?

CLAUDIA: (She nods in agreement.)

BOYNE: See, hypnosis is the most misunderstood subject. Do you know why?

CLAUDIA: (She shakes her head negatively.)

BOYNE: It's very dramatic in novels and movies that show hypnosis. You just hypnotize them and tell them to go steal the crown jewels.

CLAUDIA: They always do something weird actually.

BOYNE: Yes.

CLAUDIA: Ah, yeah.

BOYNE: And it only takes a few seconds to hypnotize anyone.

CLAUDIA: (In a serious tone) I guess, I hope, maybe, I'll be able to come out of it, won't I?

BOYNE: Well, I'll tell you what we do if you don't wake up!

CLAUDIA: (She looks scared.)

BOYNE: I have a building down in the City of Industry. It's actually a warehouse. I've got 4,000 bodies stored there.

CLAUDIA: Oh great!

BOYNE: They're all people that didn't come out of trance.

CLAUDIA: Marvelous. You're giving me a lot of confidence.

BOYNE: Yes. I tell you that so you can understand if anyone failed to come out of a trance, it would be in the headlines for ever and ever, wouldn't it?

CLAUDIA: Yes, that's true.

BOYNE: As hypnosis is a natural state of mind, you would terminate it naturally if you didn't spontaneously respond to my signal to terminate. If for some reason I left you alone, within a few minutes you'd terminate it on your own.

CLAUDIA: Yeah, yeah. (She is moving around in her chair very nervously.)

BOYNE: If you were very, very sleepy, you might sleep a half hour or an hour.

CLAUDIA: Oh.

BOYNE: But when you're asleep, you're not hypnotized.

CLAUDIA: Oh, I see.

BOYNE: Do you see the difference?

CLAUDIA: Uh-huh.

BOYNE: In hypnosis what we're talking about is the sleep of the nervous system.

CLAUDIA: How does that help you find something?

BOYNE: Because right now every time you think about that lost diamond you develop a state of tension, and tension inhibits performance.

CLAUDIA: Now, tension from what? Just because I misplaced it?

BOYNE: You said it's a valuable item, didn't you?

CLAUDIA: Yeah. I probably left it, I think, in my car, and I took my car to be fixed.

BOYNE: Yes. If you could see your face when you said, "I probably," and you began to frown. You became tense and self-critical when thinking about it. "How could I do it this way?" I heard you criticizing yourself when you said, "My husband said, 'Put it in the safe deposit box.' And I said, 'No, I'll hide it.'" And you had a critical look on your face right then.

CLAUDIA: Oh, did I? (She laughs.)

BOYNE: Yes.

CLAUDIA: Yeah, well, I guess I was right.

BOYNE: I could tell you were criticizing yourself and you were saying, "I did the wrong thing," or "I was dumb," or "Why didn't I do it his way?" Weren't you?

CLAUDIA: Well, yeah. That's what everyone says.

BOYNE: Sure.

CLAUDIA: They think I'm really flighty. Just because I misplaced something.

BOYNE: Are you flighty?

CLAUDIA: No, not really.

BOYNE: I don't get that impression.

CLAUDIA: No, no, but just because you misplace it, you know, you kind of—

BOYNE: I have misplaced things.

CLAUDIA: I know—I guess everyone does occasionally.

BOYNE: But I found them later.

CLAUDIA: Yeah. I might find it, you never know, twenty years from now.

BOYNE: You have a funny sense of humor.

CLAUDIA: (Laughter.) Do I?

BOYNE: You have kind of a comic style. You make people laugh a lot.

CLAUDIA: (She shakes her head negatively.)

BOYNE: No?

CLAUDIA: I just amuse myself.

BOYNE: Okay. That's one person you make laugh.

CLAUDIA: (She nods in agreement.)

BOYNE: Nothing wrong with that.

CLAUDIA: (She is making nervous gestures with her hands and arms.)

BOYNE: Instead of saying to me, "I'm nervous," which really means excitement of the nervous system, say to me, "I feel excited."

CLAUDIA: Oh, I feel excited?

BOYNE: Again.

CLAUDIA: I feel excited. (She begins to laugh.)

BOYNE: That's the truth, isn't it?

CLAUDIA: Well, maybe. I don't know.

BOYNE: You said you're nervous. That's what nervous is, excitement.

CLAUDIA: Is it really? Oh.

BOYNE: Right now you're being a little bit arch or playing a little bit dumb or that's the way you behave when you feel tense.

CLAUDIA: Probably it's the way I behave.

BOYNE: Because the one thing I know about you is you're really a very bright person.

CLAUDIA: Well, I don't know about that. (She almost whispers those words and waves her hand back and forth as if to say "could be.") Sometimes.

BOYNE: Are you ready for me to hypnotize you?

CLAUDIA: Yeah, if you want. (She has a scared look on her face.) That's why I'm here, isn't it?

BOYNE: That's the right answer: "That's why I'm here." Now if you'll take off your glasses.

CLAUDIA: Oh, gosh.

BOYNE: Give them to me, and I'll put them in a safe place.

CLAUDIA: They're my defense.

BOYNE: Say that again.

CLAUDIA: I hide behind them.

BOYNE: What do you hide behind the glasses?

CLAUDIA: I don't know, just things.

BOYNE: Yes.

CLAUDIA: Like I feel safe behind them.

BOYNE: Safe from?

CLAUDIA: Whatever.

BOYNE: Yes. Glasses do have a personality and do have shapes, sizes, and colors, and you have a pretty, stylish ones with red—

CLAUDIA: Kind of clashes though, doesn't it? (She says this as she looks at her blue dress.)

BOYNE: You look quite different without your glasses.

CLAUDIA: Oh, yeah. Maybe. I can never see what I actually look like. (She laughs.)

BOYNE: Are you nearsighted? Myopic?

CLAUDIA: Yeah, I was trying to figure it out.

BOYNE: So you were recently married, and this is your first marriage.

CLAUDIA: Uh-huh.

BOYNE: March, April, just a few months. How do you like married life by now?

CLAUDIA: Oh, it's interesting.

(Laugher from both Gil and Claudia.)

BOYNE: We're going to stand up. I'm going to hypnotize you standing up, but don't be concerned. You won't fall down. I'll see to that, all right?

CLAUDIA: Okay.

(Both Gil and Claudia stand up.)

BOYNE: Turn and face me. Now take one step forward.

CLAUDIA: All right.

BOYNE: Pull your feet. Let your arms hang limply by your side. SLEEP! Turn loose. Relax. Let a good, pleasant feeling come all across your body. Let each muscle and nerve grow loose and limp and as you laugh, you relax even more. Let your head begin to rotate. (Gil has his left hand on the back of Claudia's neck and his right hand on her forehead.) You can smile or laugh and it will help you relax as much as you need to, as much as you want to.

Ten, nine, eight, you're drifting down. Seven, six, five, muscles relaxing all through your neck. Four, calmly, quietly, easily, and gently relaxing even more. Three, when I use the word *sleep,* I don't mean the kind of sleep that you sleep at night. I am referring to a very pleasant state of mental and physical relaxation you're beginning to experience at this very moment. Number two, on the next number, I'll say the words "sleep deeply." When I do, you'll then be aware that you're very deeply relaxed. You're fully aware of what's going on and you're even able to think thoughts and to hear everything around you, and yet in this standing position you're more relaxed than you thought you could be. All right. Number one, just sleep deeply. (Gil snaps his fingers and pulls Claudia's head on his chest.)

Let your arms now grow limp, just like a rag doll. (Gil pulls Claudia's arms out and lets them come back to her body limply.) That's it. Just like two pieces of rope hanging from your shoulders. Just drop limply down, loosely, limply relaxing. Listen very carefully now. (Gil has his left hand on Claudia's neck and his right hand on Claudia's forehead as he says) I want you to roll your eyeballs up as if you were looking up through the inside of your skull and out a hole in the center of your forehead. Turn them right up now. Roll them up. No, imagine you're looking up, right up through the top of your head. Right through the ceiling. Right up into the sky, and you see the full moon there. It's in the evening. There's the full moon. Now I want you to look at the face of the man in the moon and as you do (Gil snaps his fingers) your eyelids lock so tightly closed (Gil taps the top of Claudia's head) the more you try to open them, the tighter they're locking closed. Make a try and satisfy yourself. They're indeed locked tightly closed. Now stop trying and relax. (Gil snaps his fingers and pulls Claudia's head on his chest.) And just sleep deeply.

You see, the first test to indicate that your subconscious is open is the ability to control your muscles through suggestion, and that's what you've just experienced and that experience is helpful for you to begin to understand what a trance is.

I want you now to raise both of your arms out in front of you. That's it. Bring the palms of your hands together, and I want you to interlock your fingers. Stiffen your arms, lock your elbows. Squeeze your fingers now very tightly against the back of your hands. That's it. Lock your elbows and squeeze those fingers very tight. Tighter. Much tighter than that. That's it. Lock them out. Now you're getting it. Very stiff. Very tight. Very rigid. Hold them very tightly together. (Gil is standing behind Claudia tapping her forehead as he is giving these instructions and now pulls her back against him.) That's it. (Gil pulls Claudia's head back against his chest and says) Imagine your two hands are carved of one solid block of wood. They're locked so tightly closed. The more you try to pull your hands apart, the tighter they're locking closed. Try now to pull your hands apart and find them stuck tight. Make a try to satisfy yourself. When you're satisfied, say aloud the words, "I'm satisfied." (Gil is tapping Claudia's forehead with his finger.) Say aloud the words.

CLAUDIA: I'm satisfied.

BOYNE: All right. Now I'm going to count to three. Open your eyes, try to pull your hands apart, and your hands are stuck. No matter what you do or say or think, they remain stuck until I release them. (Gil taps Claudia's forehead and says) Open your eyes and look at your hands. Try to pull them apart and they're stuck tighter and tighter. And when you're absolutely convinced that they're stuck, say out loud, "They're stuck."

CLAUDIA: They're stuck.

BOYNE: (Gil snaps his fingers and places his hand on Claudia's forehead and says) Close your eyelids down. Let your eyelids close down, and I'll touch your hands. They begin to relax. Relax your arms. That's it. Now slowly pull your hands apart. Let them drop limply to your side and relax even more.

CLAUDIA: Ouch!

BOYNE: That's it. (Gil moves in front of Claudia again and places his left hand on the back of her neck and his right hand on her forehead rocking it.) Now you just said "ouch." What is it that's causing you to say "ouch"?

CLAUDIA: I feel so funny.

BOYNE: You feel funny.

CLAUDIA: Uh-huh.

BOYNE: And?

CLAUDIA: And my hands...

BOYNE: Strange.

CLAUDIA: Yeah, my hands.

BOYNE: Tell me about the strangeness. Is it a tingling in your finger tips?

CLAUDIA: My hands.

BOYNE: That's part of the sensation of hypnosis as you relax. I'm going to take you one step forward. Take a step forward. Now I'm going to turn you with your legs back up against your couch. When I push you down into the couch, you'll sit down.

CLAUDIA: Uh-huh.

BOYNE: And you'll go much deeper into this pleasant, relaxed state.

CLAUDIA: (She groans.)

BOYNE: All right. Here you go. One, two, three. Bend your knees and down. (Claudia sits down on couch.) That's it. Now you're relaxing more than before. I want you now to just let your mind relax. Separate your knees. That's it. Let your arms relax. Now listen very carefully.

I'm going to count from one up to twenty, and as I do, a light, easy, pleasant sensation moves into your right hand and into your right arm. As I continue counting, that feeling grows stronger and stronger. Soon you'll feel the first slight movements, slight movement of the fingers, a twitching of the muscles. Then your hand begins to lift (Gil places his little finger under Claudia's hand and lifts her hand and arm in demonstration.) Your arm begins to lift and it continues moving, lifting, and rising until it comes to rest over on your body. Now when you feel that movement in your hand and in your arm, don't try to resist. You could resist if you chose to, that's not why you're here. Let your subconscious mind do its perfect work.

All right. We're ready to begin. Number one. The first light, easy sensation moves into the finger tips of your right hand. Number two. The feeling is spreading around beneath the fingernails. On number three, it's moving up to the first joint of the fingers. Number four, spreading over across the back of the hand. Number five. Now moving into the thumb. On number six, you're left hand begins to feel heavy. While on number seven, your right hand is feeling lighter and lighter with each number I count. Number eight, the light sensation is spreading through the palm of your hand now and moving up toward your wrist. On number nine, your left hand is growing heavier and heavier while your right hand grows lighter and lighter with each number I count. Number ten. It's up to the wrist from the finger tips. All the way up to the wrist your hand has grown light, light and free, just as light as a feather floating in the breeze and even lighter, as light as a gas filled balloon. Just as a gas filled balloon will rise and float toward the ceiling, in the same way you're right hand is ready to begin moving, lifting, rising, and floating, coming up and moving up until it comes to rest up upon your body.

(Claudia moves her right hand up and then places it back down on her lap.)

Eleven, think of your left hand again.

CLAUDIA: No, I'm asleep.

BOYNE: That's right, and your left hand feels different. Your left hand feels heavier. While on number twelve, your right hand grows lighter and lighter. And as it begins (Gil puts his little finger up under Claudia's right hand) just let it continue moving and lifting and rising, and you'll find it is quite easy for you to do. Number thirteen. That light sensation spreads up your arm. Let your hand continue moving and lifting and rising. (Claudia laughs.) It seems strange, yet it's strange and pleasant. On number fourteen, let it continue and feel how heavy that left hand feels, like it's made of lead. Fifteen. Your right hand is light all the way up to your elbow and it's moving up in toward your body, in toward your chest. Sixteen, spreading up toward your shoulder. Seventeen. When your hand touches your body, you'll find that you're twice as relaxed as you are right now. Eighteen. Coming right in toward your body. Nineteen. Let it drop right up on your chest. (Claudia's hand touches her chest.) Number twenty. And as it drops on your chest, you find that you're more relaxed than you were just a few moments ago. Now your left arm feels as though it were made of marble or stone or lead. Your left arm feels so heavy that just the thought of lifting it seems more than you want to concern yourself with at this time. You may wish to make an effort to lift your left arm, but it seems like it's more than you want to bother with. All right. You can stop trying.

The feeling that you felt as your right arm felt light and was lifting, that's the feeling of hypnosis. The feeling that you felt as your left arm felt heavy, that's the feeling of hypnosis. The feeling that you felt as your eyelids stuck is the feeling of hypnosis. And the feeling that you felt as your hands were stuck together is the feeling of hypnosis. We call these responses the feeling of hypnosis because you know intellectually, just as I do, there's no reason for one hand to feel lighter than the other hand or for the left hand to feel heavier than the right. They should always feel the same. There's no reason for your eyelids not to open the instant you think about opening them, and there's no rational, intellectual reason for your hands not to come apart the moment you make the effort. What has happened is that the part of your mind that reasons rationally and intellectually just relaxes. It doesn't disappear. It's as if it sits off in an easy chair and watches everything taking place, so that you become aware of two parts of your mind operating at the same time. If you understand what I've said and you're aware of that, nod your head.

CLAUDIA: (She nods in agreement.)

BOYNE: Fine. As excited as you were a few moments ago, you can find that inner excitement becoming quieter and calmer with each passing moment. If you're aware that inner excitement is becoming quieter and calmer with each passing moment, just nod your head.

CLAUDIA: (She nods in agreement.)

BOYNE: Fine. You see when we talk about the relaxation or sleep of the nervous system, that's what hypnosis truly is. Now there's another very beneficial part of hypnosis—because your mind relaxes, it's able to do more for you. You know any time you've tried to remember something, maybe a person's name or an address, and you say, "Well, their address is, now wait a minute, I'll think of it. Now wait, wait," and the harder you try, the more difficult it becomes. But the moment you say, "Oh, well, it will come to me," then in a minute or two or three it comes to you. If you ever had that kind of experience, just nod your head.

CLAUDIA: (She nods in agreement.)

BOYNE: Fine. When something is lost that has an emotional significance because it's valuable or important or in some way emotionally meaningful, even though one can afford the loss and the value might be purely sentimental, or it might have been business papers, a contract, or whatever, there's always tension that is generated. And when you try to think about it, your mind doesn't function properly and your memory doesn't serve you properly because of the anxiety. If you understand that nod your head.

CLAUDIA: (She nods in agreement.)

BOYNE: Now in this relaxed state, you can remember vividly. Now, for example, when I count from three down to one, I want you to go back to breakfast this morning, if you ate breakfast, or if not, to your first meal of the day. (As Gil counts, he taps Claudia's forehead.) One, two, three. Now you're back to your very first meal of today which is Friday. I want you to tell me about it.

CLAUDIA: What do you want to know?

BOYNE: Are you eating alone or are you with someone?

CLAUDIA: I'm with David.

BOYNE: David is your husband?

CLAUDIA: (She nods in agreement.)

BOYNE: Good. What is it that you're eating?

CLAUDIA: He made fried eggs.

BOYNE: I want you to speak in the present tense as if you are right there.

CLAUDIA: Oh, okay. Fried eggs.

BOYNE: All right. And do you have anything else with your fried eggs?

CLAUDIA: Toast and coffee.

BOYNE: How's your coffee this morning?

CLAUDIA: It's okay.

BOYNE: Now here's what I want you to do. I'll count from three down to one, and we're going back to last Sunday, five days ago. Three, two, one. (Gil taps Claudia's forehead as he counts.) It's Sunday now. Is it in the morning, afternoon or evening? Pick one. Quickly.

CLAUDIA: Afternoon.

BOYNE: It's in the afternoon on Sunday, and are you alone or is someone with you?

CLAUDIA: David.

BOYNE: Are you indoors or outside?

CLAUDIA: Indoors.

BOYNE: What's going on? What are you two doing?

CLAUDIA: Sunday, movies.

BOYNE: You're getting ready to go to the movies or you're watching movies on your video?

CLAUDIA: Going to the movies.

BOYNE: Going to the movies. What have you decided to go see?

CLAUDIA: *Gotcha.*

BOYNE: All right. Fine. Let your mind grow clear. (As Gil says this, he places his hand on Claudia's forehead.) Now this time, I'm going to count from ten down to one, and we're going right back to a time when you're opening a package, a box, and there's some costume jewelry, and that's where you've hidden the diamond. Ten, nine, eight, seven, six, five, four, three, two, one. (Gil taps Claudia's forehead as he counts.) Now you've opened the file cabinet and what are you doing?

CLAUDIA: I'm looking for the little tin box, and I take it out.

BOYNE: Now you've got the tin box.

CLAUDIA: Uh-huh. And I put it in my purse.

BOYNE: You're putting it in your purse. Have you opened it at all?

CLAUDIA: Yeah.

BOYNE: Describe that. "I take it out. Now I'm opening it."

CLAUDIA: I'm opening it and I take a look. And the diamond necklace is wrapped in tissue paper.

BOYNE: You see the tissue paper there?

CLAUDIA: Uh-huh. I unwrap it and there it is, and I wrap it up again and close the little tin box.

BOYNE: Now the box is going into your purse.

CLAUDIA: Uh-huh.

BOYNE: As I tap your forehead, you begin moving forward in time from the time that you've put this tin box into your purse. (Gil taps Claudia's forehead.) Just give a report.

CLAUDIA: After I put it in my purse, I leave David's office and I go to my flat, and I start packing things away.

BOYNE: You're at the flat. Which room are you in?

CLAUDIA: My bedroom.

BOYNE: In your bedroom, and what are you doing there?

CLAUDIA: I'm looking around the bedroom.

BOYNE: Where is your purse?

CLAUDIA: In the bedroom, on the bed.

BOYNE: Have you opened it and taken out the tin box, or is the box still inside the purse?

CLAUDIA: It's still inside.

BOYNE: Now, you've decided to pack some things, is that it?

CLAUDIA: (She nods in agreement.)

BOYNE: All right. Are you packing them in boxes?

CLAUDIA: (She nods in agreement.)

BOYNE: What are you going to pack first?

CLAUDIA: I go to the closet. I'm at the closet and I'm just kind of looking at the mess.

BOYNE: Trying to figure out where to start.

CLAUDIA: Yeah, and I guess I start. I get a box up from the floor and I just start filling it with some of the drawers in the closet—all the things—and then I think I open my purse.

BOYNE: I want you to leave out the words "I think."

CLAUDIA: Okay. All I know is I—

BOYNE: I don't want you to think or remember. I just want you to be there. Give a report. You don't have to see it clearly in your mind. Just keep speaking.

CLAUDIA: I go to my purse and I remember someone told me that when they were robbed that they didn't take their money because they put it with a bunch of open letters and bills. So I go to my bookshelf where I keep my bills, and I put the tin little box there and cover it up, and I continue to pack.

BOYNE: Now say again, "It's on the bookshelf."

CLAUDIA: It's on the bookshelf where the letters are.

BOYNE: Where you keep your bills. Now, are the bills just laying there or—

CLAUDIA: They're stacked.

BOYNE: Are they in a box or any—

CLAUDIA: Loose. It's a high stack actually, I'd say five inches.

BOYNE: You have a lot of bills.

CLAUDIA: And letters.

BOYNE: Now you take the tin box, and put it behind the stack, is that right?

CLAUDIA: Uh-huh.

BOYNE: And now?

CLAUDIA: And just continue to put clothes in the boxes and shoes and whatnot, and then I go to my car and I drive my car around because my files are at the backdoor.

BOYNE: Say, "I'm at the backdoor." You drive your car from the front to the back.

CLAUDIA: To the back and then I start putting boxes in the car.

BOYNE: Continue.

CLAUDIA: And then I leave.

BOYNE: Now you're ready to start your car and leave.

CLAUDIA: (She nods in agreement.)

BOYNE: You recall now that you left the tin box up behind the bills, behind the stack of bills?

CLAUDIA: (She nods in agreement.)

BOYNE: When I tap your forehead we'll move ahead in time now until when you're concerning yourself with the tin box. (Gil taps Claudia's forehead.)

CLAUDIA: I'm in my apartment again and I'm packing up the bookshelf this time. I'm putting all the boxes and papers and whatnot in boxes.

BOYNE: Yes.

CLAUDIA: But I don't recall the tin box being there.

BOYNE: No. Don't try to recall. Just do it.

CLAUDIA: Oh.

BOYNE: You're picking up the boxes, putting them in boxes. Now you come to the stack of bills and letters.

CLAUDIA: Right. That's in a separate box, all that junk, and I don't know if the box is still there.

BOYNE: Is it there or is it not there?

CLAUDIA: Oh, it is.

BOYNE: All right.

CLAUDIA: And I put it in my purse.

BOYNE: So now it's back in your purse.

CLAUDIA: (She nods in agreement.)

BOYNE: All right. That's very good.

CLAUDIA: And I—(Laughter) Do you want to know more?

BOYNE: Sure. Just keep reporting.

CLAUDIA: I think I leave some—

BOYNE: Don't think.

CLAUDIA: I'm trying, oh, okay. I'm there. What am I doing?

BOYNE: You've just taken the box and you've put it in your purse.

CLAUDIA: Right.

BOYNE: Now what about these boxes and things you've packed up? Are you going to carry them out now?

CLAUDIA: Well, some I do and some I don't because they're heavy. So I just take a few of them and do the same number, put my car in the back.

BOYNE: Do you keep your car keys in your purse?

CLAUDIA: Uh-huh.

BOYNE: Your purse is with you?

CLAUDIA: Right.

BOYNE: Because you're going to start the car.

CLAUDIA: Right. And I go to David's house, and I unload the books in the living room and—

BOYNE: You come in with a box of books.

CLAUDIA: Uh-huh, and my purse.

BOYNE: And your purse. Put them down.

CLAUDIA: Uh-huh.

BOYNE: All right. See your purse where ever you set it.

CLAUDIA: In the family room.

BOYNE: And now?

CLAUDIA: And now I put the boxes in the living room and then, I don't know. I can't recall.

BOYNE: When I count to three a thought will come to your mind. One, two, three. (Gil places his hand on Claudia's head.) Quickly now, speak.

CLAUDIA: Yeah.

BOYNE: Let it come out.

CLAUDIA: It can't.

BOYNE: Yes. I'm going to count to three. When I tap your forehead, I'm going to ask you a question. The answer will come out by spelling. One, two, three. (Gil is tapping Claudia's forehead and saying) Quickly now, a word, a letter. The first letter is, let it come out. A letter of the alphabet. Quickly. Let it come out.

CLAUDIA: Nothing is coming.

BOYNE: Speak a letter of the alphabet. A letter.

CLAUDIA: B.

BOYNE: The next. Quickly, speak.

CLAUDIA: A.

BOYNE: The next. Quickly. Speak now in a hurry.

CLAUDIA: In a hurry?

BOYNE: Yes.

CLAUDIA: T.

BOYNE: Okay, and the next.

CLAUDIA: H.

BOYNE: And the next.

CLAUDIA: R.

BOYNE: And the next.

CLAUDIA: O.

BOYNE: And the next.

CLAUDIA: O.

BOYNE: And the next.

CLAUDIA: M.

BOYNE: Now I'm going to tap your forehead. I want a phrase or a sentence or two that uses the word *bathroom* in this connection. Quickly. Speak.

CLAUDIA: What was that again? You want a sentence, bathroom. Maybe I went to the bathroom.

BOYNE: Yes.

CLAUDIA: With the diamond.

BOYNE: Yes.

CLAUDIA: I went to the bathroom with the diamond.

BOYNE: Now you're in the bathroom.

CLAUDIA: How weird!

BOYNE: With the diamond. Now what are you going to do? Are you going to clean it, wash it, or what are you going to do in the bathroom with it? Hide it?

CLAUDIA: Probably.

BOYNE: Are you going to hide it?

CLAUDIA: I hid it, yes.

BOYNE: "I hid it in the bathroom."

CLAUDIA: There's oodles of drawers there.

BOYNE: Okay.

CLAUDIA: So I must—

BOYNE: "I hid it in the bathroom." Now, one more time.

CLAUDIA: Uh-huh.

BOYNE: This time I'm going to tap your forehead.

CLAUDIA: Oh, oh.

BOYNE: Once again we're going to do it by spelling a word that will link you to where you put it in the bathroom.

Ready. One, two, three. (Gil taps Claudia's forehead and then opens her mouth and says) A letter, a letter. Speak quickly. Let it out. It out now. Quickly. A letter. Quickly.

CLAUDIA: Okay.

BOYNE: Quickly.

CLAUDIA: A letter.

BOYNE: Yes. Any letter.

CLAUDIA: S.

BOYNE: S. Quickly. Don't think about it. Let it come out. Your subconscious produces it. Right now, right now, quickly.

CLAUDIA: S.

BOYNE: Yeah.

CLAUDIA: S-E.

BOYNE: Yes.

CLAUDIA: L.

BOYNE: The next.

CLAUDIA: F.

BOYNE: Self.

CLAUDIA: Self, how weird!

BOYNE: When you look in the mirror, what do you see?

CLAUDIA: Myself.

BOYNE: Yes.

CLAUDIA: Laughter.

BOYNE: Is it near the mirror?

CLAUDIA: Oh, yeah. (Claudia sounds amazed.)

BOYNE: What is it that is near the mirror?

CLAUDIA: There's two mirrors, or three actually, and one side it has little shelves, the other side it has little shelves and the medicine cabinet.

BOYNE: One more time when I count to three, a thought will come to your mind. It quickly has to do with looking in the mirror and the shelves and the medicine chest. One, two, three. (Gil puts his hand on Claudia's head.) Speak now. Speak it out.

CLAUDIA: I can't.

BOYNE: Let a sentence come out. Speak now!

CLAUDIA: It's by the bathtub.

BOYNE: All right. It's by the bathtub. Now when I tap your forehead, I want you to see the spot. One, two, three. (Gil is tapping Claudia's forehead.) Speak now!

CLAUDIA: It's in the left-hand shelf. It's the little one, I think.

BOYNE: All right. Now I want you to take a deep breath and for the moment just let your mind relax. Let all the tensions concerned with this just drain from your body.

CLAUDIA: Uh-huh.

BOYNE: Feel good now?

CLAUDIA: Uh-huh.

BOYNE: Thank the Greater Intelligence for allowing your memory to work for you perfectly.

CLAUDIA: Uh-huh.

BOYNE: You must feel relieved and happy.

CLAUDIA: Uh-huh.

BOYNE: You know just what you're going to do now, don't you?

CLAUDIA: Uh-huh.

BOYNE: All right. Fine. Before I get you up, is there anything further you want to say to me or ask me or tell me?

CLAUDIA: Thank you.

BOYNE: Quickly, who do I remind you of?

CLAUDIA: A doctor.

BOYNE: A doctor. How am I like a doctor?

CLAUDIA: Laughter.

BOYNE: Because I know what goes on inside you?

CLAUDIA: (She nods in agreement while she is still laughing.) You're trustworthy.

BOYNE: Trustworthy. Good. I'm going to count to five. On the count of five, eyelids open, fully aware with a full conscious memory of everything that you've experienced, everything that's passed through your mind. One. Slowly, calmly, easily, and gently returning to your full awareness once again. Two. Each muscle and nerve in your body is loose and limp and relaxed. You feel good. Three. From head to toe, you're feeling perfect in every way. On number four, your eyes begin to feel sparkling clear. On the next number now, eyelids open, fully aware, feeling wonderfully good. Number five, eyelids open now. Take a deep breath. Fill up your lungs and stretch.

CLAUDIA: (She opens her eyes and has a very happy look about her face.)

BOYNE: Well, you kind of surprised yourself, didn't you?

CLAUDIA: (She nods in agreement and smiles.) Yeah. Gosh.

BOYNE: Tell me about it.

CLAUDIA: Well, I found—it's in the bathroom. Amazing. I don't remember doing that at all. How weird.

BOYNE: (Laughs.)

CLAUDIA: It's really weird. Gosh, I feel hot.

BOYNE: Yes. It's hot. I want to tell you something. Look at me. This is off the record.

CLAUDIA: What?

BOYNE: This is just for you.

CLAUDIA: What?

BOYNE: You're a very pretty woman, but somewhere you decided that you'd be safer to play clown. Look at me. You make a lot of funny faces, a lot of funny gestures and—

CLAUDIA: Oh, I learned that in school.

BOYNE: And you roll your eyes a lot, and it may be cute, but I don't know if cute is the way that you might want to be defined. You're a married lady now and growing up.

CLAUDIA: (She nods in agreement.)

BOYNE: Maybe you prefer to be seen as elegant, beautiful.

CLAUDIA: Elegant, I don't know. I can't picture that.

BOYNE: Lovely?

CLAUDIA: No.

BOYNE: Is it time to start picturing those things?

CLAUDIA: Maybe, I don't know. I always goof up when I try to be that way.

BOYNE: Will you promise me you'll try more often?

CLAUDIA: Okay. Sure.

BOYNE: Whether or not you goof up.

CLAUDIA: Okay.

BOYNE: I've enjoyed being here with you.

CLAUDIA: Thank you.

BOYNE: There's one more thing. After you go home and find the diamond, please call me and tell me about it.

CLAUDIA: Okay. Okay. Ciao. Oh, I'm so hot.

BOYNE: The function of stimulating memory recall is really quite easy. Over the years I've helped people find business contracts, including one that was for the sale of a chain of grocery stores, and it would be quite expensive if the papers had not been found. I had another case of an expensive piece of jewelry that disappeared that had been given to a woman by her lover. I worked with her and she didn't get any results, but from the start I felt that the expensive jewelry had not been lost, but had been disposed of in some other way, and I felt certain that this lady knew the disposal of that item, but she was not going to reveal it. Her life would have been in great jeopardy if she had.

There's a feeling that comes to you when you can see the subconscious mind at work as you saw it here, and other times when you know the person is just determined to conceal the truth about what happened. In more than a hundred instances of helping people to find lost items or to remember ideas or memories that they want to recall, I have been successful more than 80 percent of the time. Don't hesitate to work with a person and to help them find lost items and lost memories.

Until the next time, this is Gil Boyne.

(Less than forty-five minutes later, Claudia called to breathlessly announce that she had found the necklace.)

HYPNOTHERAPY TO DEVELOP SELF-ESTEEM AND TO OVERCOME ALCOHOLISM

The Case of Bud ("Born to Lose")

A depressed male, sixty-one years old, is convinced that he is a loser in life. He suffers from alcoholism, insomnia, low self-esteem, self-isolation, and negative thinking.

In two one-hour sessions on consecutive days, Bud experiences an amazing personal transformation.

Filmed before a hypnotherapy class of thirty-five professionals in Chicago, these sessions demonstrate age regression, abreaction, Gestalt dialogues, and many of Gil Boyne's original uncovering/reprogramming techniques.

THE CASE OF BUD
"Born to Lose"
Session One

(The Setting: A Hypnotherapy Class in Chicago)

(BOYNE ADDRESSES THE AUDIENCE)

BOYNE: Hello. This is Gil Boyne, and welcome again to the Hypnotherapy Video Clinic. Today we're starting a new case history. Our client today is Bud. Let's meet him now.

(BOYNE ADDRESSES BUD)

Bud, welcome.

BUD: Thank you.

BOYNE: You're here from Wisconsin.

BUD: Correct.

BOYNE: How can I help you today?

BUD: (Bud has a hangdog expression on his face and looks sad and depressed.) Well, I need help in several areas. I need self-confidence. I have a loss of memory. I can't seem to remember anything. Seems like I need help in just about every area. I can't sing. I can't dance. I do everything wrong.

BOYNE: Can't even whistle, huh?

BUD: No, I can't.

BOYNE: There was an old vaudeville gag. It went, "I can't sing and I can't dance, but I sure can make love." How did you first learn of me?

BUD: I got your catalog through the mail. I wrote you a letter, you answered the letter, and I called you and you invited me to come here.

BOYNE: I told you that I would be coming to Chicago in April. I said if you'd come to Chicago, I would work with you and here we are. Now you said, "I have no confidence." Was that your statement?

BUD: Yes.

BOYNE: I'm going to give you a choice. Is it, "I have no confidence" or "I've lost my confidence" or "I never had any confidence," or some other statement?

BUD: I've never had any confidence.

BOYNE: Wrong! You came into the world loaded with confidence. When you lay in your crib and your diaper was wet and you were hungry, you made a loud noise and someone came and took care of it, and that increased your confidence. Some people go through their lifetime and never learn any other method for getting what they want. They just keep making a loud noise until someone comes and takes care of it.

BUD: (He nods in agreement.)

BOYNE: Do you know someone like that?

BUD: (Laughs) I suppose I do.

BOYNE: I'm going to propose to you that that early confidence that you had is still with you. I'd like you to think back for just a minute when you were maybe four or five years old—you sprang out of bed about five o'clock in the morning and your imagination was excited with your plans for all the things that you were going to do that day, and obstacles just didn't exist, or if they did, in your imagination you just swept them away. You had then what's been called "the most precious gift of the mind," a belief in yourself. If you had it then, what's happened to it? A rule of physics is that you can't create energy, nor can you destroy it, you can only transform it. There was no one around you wise enough to protect that precious gift of your mind and it became transformed. You were told what you couldn't do, what you shouldn't do, and what your limitations and restrictions were, and now you're loaded with confidence. You're confident that you can't remember things.

BUD: (He nods in agreement.)

BOYNE: You just told me that with great confidence, didn't you?

BUD: I sure did.

BOYNE: You're confident that you're a washout in life, aren't you?

BUD: I am.

BOYNE: You're totally confident in your belief that you can't have a good love relationship and you have a full investment of confidence in all of those vile, negative beliefs about yourself, don't you, Bud?

BUD: I do.

BOYNE: So you really haven't lost anything, you've just transformed it. What's your response to that?

BUD: I don't feel anything.

BOYNE: That's a different kind of response, "I'm cut off from myself."

BUD: I'm a firm believer that I just can't do anything right. I'll goof it up, just give me time.

BOYNE: I want to talk to the class for just a moment. (Gil puts his hand on Bud's arm and turns and addresses the class.) If you just listen to the client, you get such a wealth of information, sentence by sentence. I'm being overwhelmed with information. "I just can't feel anything." What does that mean? "I cut off my feelings because if I let my feelings be open and available to me, I might make contact with a certain kind of feeling that I avoid because it's too painful." I set that aside in my mind and I ask, "intense fear of rejection, powerful feelings of being unloved?" I put a question mark because I am not saying this is a fact. I say, "Let's keep examining the evidence."

The next statements are "I'm just utterly convinced that I can't do anything right. I'm bound to louse it up. I have a powerfully intense fear of criticism," and you begin to see how you get the information, sentence by sentence, and you get it all within the first ten minutes. You get ninety percent of what is most significant. Everything else that emerges confirms and corroborates everything you've already gotten. (Gil turns to Bud and addresses him.) Please continue. The last thing you said was that you're utterly convinced that you can't do anything right. You even said that with a note of pride in your voice.

BUD: (Laughter) Well, I didn't mean it that way.

BOYNE: It came out that way. Please continue.

BUD: Well, it just seems that every time I try anything, it just never comes out right.

BOYNE: That song is "Born to Lose."

BUD: Well, I suppose they wrote it for me.

BOYNE: (Gil taps Bud's arm as he chuckles and says) At least you've sung it a lot, haven't you?

BUD: (Laughter) All my life.

BOYNE: Sure. (Gil places his hand on Bud's arm and turns to the class and addresses the class) "All my life," that's a feeling. "It ain't necessarily so," says the song, but he feels that it is so. (Gil turns back to address Bud.) All right, Bud. Continue.

BUD: Well, I just don't feel any different now at my age than I did when I was just a little fellow.

BOYNE: Now what does that mean? Earlier today we worked with another man who said when he speaks to people, quite often he feels that he's small and they're large because of his stuttering problem in the past. Is that something like what you're feeling right now?

BUD: I suppose it is. It's—I just feel that everybody has more to offer. They're smarter than I am. They're better talkers than I am. They're better doers.

BOYNE: Sure. (Gil turns and addresses the class.) There are two major attitudes, one at each end of a continuum. One is that the universe is intrinsically malevolent and evil, and it's characterized by negative beliefs about oneself: "I'm never able to do anything right, I'm not smart," and so on, and then confirmed by reasons which are called alibis: "If only I had a better education; If only my mother had loved me more than she loved my brother; If only I had married a different woman; If only I had been born with a different skin color; If only I had been born in a different country, a different city." You name it, the list is endless. By the way, when that attitude overwhelms us, it is labeled "paranoia." "They're out to get me. They're conspiring against me. The FBI has my house wired." The opposite attitude is, "All that I require for the fulfillment of my deepest needs and the realization of my potential exists for me now."

I don't set a goal for Bud and say, "I'm going to move you from point A to point B," but I do say, "We've got to move him from where he is now and toward a new place where he can experience life more fully." Then he can realize that even at age sixty there may be twenty or even thirty years in which he can feel differently about himself and the world around him and his capacity to relate to it in a creative way. (Gil now turns and addresses Bud.) Now that you've identified yourself as such a nothing, tell me about it!

BUD: Well, I don't like to think of myself as nothing because I've tried to better myself, but I just don't make any progress.

BOYNE: According to your history now, you've said, "I've tried and I've always failed," so I can't give you any points. You get no points for trying if you've always failed. The world measures you by what you've done, not by what you've tried to do, especially if you keep trying and never do, because trying is lying. Let me say it again. Trying is lying. Repeat after me, "Trying is lying."

BUD: Trying is lying.

BOYNE: Trying is lying because when you say, "I'll try," the word *try* incorporates the expectancy and potential for failure, doesn't it?

BUD: Yes.

BOYNE: If I threw this pencil down to the floor and I said, "Try to pick it up," and you picked it up and handed it to me and I said, "No, try to pick it up," and dropped it again and you picked it up and handed it to me, and I dropped it again and said, "Try to pick it up," about the third time you'd say, "What are you talking about; I keep picking it up." And I said, "No, try to pick it up." You'd say, "That doesn't make sense," and I say, "Of course it doesn't make sense." But if I were an orthopedic surgeon and I had completed a back surgery on you and your back had been very stiff, and we were working with therapy to loosen it up, and now I want to see how much flexibility is in your back. I'd say, "Try to pick up the pen." Then and then only would *try* have any application because *try* indicates difficulty. When an athlete says, "Today I'm going to try to set a new world record," that indicates difficulty, doesn't it?

BUD: Yes.

BOYNE: So when I say, "I don't give you points for trying," I'm really saying to you, "Stop bragging about trying and failing" because that's just your way of saying, "It's not for the lack of effort. It's not because I haven't tried. It's not because I'm lazy," while you lay by the side of the road and let life go by. "I've made efforts," but your efforts, by your testimony, have been ineffective, ineffectual, and counterproductive as well. True or false?

BUD: Well, it's not true and it's not false.

BOYNE: Then you tell me how it is.

BUD: Well, it seems as though I've done the necessary things.

BOYNE: Such as.

BUD: Built a home and I have it paid for.

BOYNE: Good.

BUD: And outside of that I have a job I've been on for thirty-five years.

BOYNE: (Gil taps Bud's arm in assurance and turns to address the class.) Now we start to get someplace because Bud just told us, "I took care of my survival needs," in a culture where it is rather easy to take care of your survival needs provided you don't listen to propaganda that says, "The government should take care of your survival needs." That means food, shelter and clothing. (Gil places his hand on Bud's arm and addresses Bud.) I talked yesterday about the fact that there is something criminal about a system that takes a marvelous organism like a human being and says that you can work for one firm or one company doing pretty much the same kind of things for thirty-five years and then gives you a gold watch and a pat on the back and you say, "Is that all there is?" Bud, is that the question you've been asking?

BUD: Yes, I guess it is.

BOYNE: All right. What do you want from me?

BUD: I want you to instill that confidence in me.

BOYNE: Give you a transfusion?

BUD: That's right.

BOYNE: I've got a big hypodermic needle over there. It's about that long... (Gil stretches his arms wide to indicate length.) It's filled with all kinds of good things that I drew out of the bottle labeled Self-Confidence.

BUD: Well, you've done marvelous things for other people.

BOYNE: (Gil taps Bud on the arm.) I helped others do wonderful things for themselves that they didn't know they could do, and you're just as blind to your own power as they were, maybe more so.

BUD: (He nods in agreement.)

BOYNE: If I had a magic wand and I waved it now and I said, "Now you can achieve whatever you want and by five o'clock this afternoon it's yours," how would your life be changed?

BUD: Well, I wish I could just go out and do all the things I'd like to do.

BOYNE: I want you to stop being vague. We're going to start right now going from the general to the specific. Tell me one thing you'd go out of here and do now that you've got it all. Boyne has waved his magic wand and said, "You've got it." What are you going to do or be or feel or experience?

BUD: I just think I'd just take off and take a long trip somewhere. Get away from everybody.

BOYNE: All right. "I would travel."

BUD: Yes.

BOYNE: What's keeping you from traveling now?

BUD: My job.

BOYNE: All right. Then if I solved whatever it is you want

solved, you wouldn't be concerned about your job anymore?

BUD: Oh, certainly I would. Sure.

BOYNE: Then you couldn't travel.

BUD: Well, not now I couldn't (laughter).

BOYNE: Listen again. I'm going over the same material again. Sometimes we develop a lifetime pattern of playing dumb because we believe that we're dumb. I don't believe that you're dumb. I think you're very intelligent. So you can stop playing dumb with me, okay?

BUD: (He nods in agreement.)

BOYNE: I know that you understand every word that I say.

BUD: Yes.

BOYNE: All right. I want you to pretend with me for a moment that I wave a magic wand, and you've got what you came for. Now you're going out of here, how is your life different than it was when you arrived?

BUD: Well, I just would feel a whole lot different if I would feel confident. I wouldn't be afraid of people. I wouldn't be afraid to speak up and say something for fear that after I said it somebody would say something that I wouldn't be able to come up with the right answer to.

BOYNE: How would your life be different?

BUD: Well, I think I would be a happy man.

BOYNE: How would your life be different?

BUD: Well, I just think I'd just do things in general.

BOYNE: Are you saying to me you don't even have a plan, an expectancy, you can't generate an image of one thing, or one form of behavior that would be different except for these abstract generalities—"I'd be happy. I'd feel better," and so on?

BUD: I suppose, yes.

BOYNE: That's pitiful! Let's go back. What is it you would like to get for yourself? What do you want from me? I want you to be as specific as you can.

BUD: Well, I'd like to be free of having all these doubts about myself. I want to be around people. I don't want to hide from them, and when there's a conversation going on, I'd like to contribute. I just don't want to stand there like a mute and just be a listener.

BOYNE: If you don't want to stand there like a mute, why do you?

BUD: I'm afraid to say things.

BOYNE: That's the right answer. Now make it a longer statement, "I'm afraid to contribute to the conversation..."

BUD: I'm afraid to contribute to the conversation because I might just—I'm afraid I'm going to make mistakes.

BOYNE: "I'm afraid I'm going to make a mistake and then..."

BUD: I'm going to be corrected.

BOYNE: "I'll be corrected or..."

BUD: Embarrassed.

BOYNE: Or, "I'll be embarrassed by my thought that they're thinking that I'm dumb."

BUD: That's right.

BOYNE: "Just like I always think about myself."

BUD: That's right.

BOYNE: Are you dumb?

BUD: Well, in my mind I really don't think so, but it seems that everything I do is dumb. I say dumb things.

BOYNE: Sure. You've learned to play dumb so well that you've become an expert.

BUD: I guess I am. (Gil shakes Bud's hand and chuckles.)

BOYNE: Well, realizing the truth is an important first step. I don't want to indicate that you sat down one day and wrote on a piece of paper, "From now on I play dumb." It started long before that.

BUD: That's right.

BOYNE: Have you ever sought help for these feelings before?

BUD: No.

BOYNE: Do you have any history of depression?

BUD: I feel like I'm depressed all the time.

BOYNE: Sure. If you're not connected to life, it's a down feeling. Have you ever taken any kind of medication for depression, tranquilizers or energizers, those kinds of things?

BUD: Yes, one time I did for high blood pressure.

BOYNE: All right. How do you get along with alcohol?

BUD: Well, it's just been the last year that I started drinking quite a bit. I used to be a social drinker.

BOYNE: I want you to tell me whether you drink beer, wine, or whiskey, and the quantity you drink daily. Is it two cans of beer, three glasses of wine, eight ounces of whiskey? Vodka, rum, gin? What is the quantity and frequency of your alcohol consumption now?

BUD: I drink brandy and I drink it straight with diet Pepsi for a wash. I consume probably eight, ten ounces a night.

BOYNE: How long have you been doing that?

BUD: A year and a half.

BOYNE: How would you feel if I told you you were an alcoholic?

BUD: I wouldn't believe you.

BOYNE: Describe to me an alcoholic as you understand the term.

BUD: Well, an alcoholic is a man that can't stop drinking. He drinks continuously, takes it to work in his lunch bucket.

BOYNE: So as long as you don't take it to work in your lunch bucket, you're not an alcoholic.

BUD: Well, some guys do, I don't. I don't have to have it all the time, but I when I'm at home by myself, I drink.

BOYNE: You live alone?

BUD: My mother lives with me.

BOYNE: Have you been married?

BUD: I married years ago.

BOYNE: Are you divorced or a widower?

BUD: Divorced.

BOYNE: Were there children from that marriage?

BUD: Yeah, there are two.

BOYNE: Are they now adults?

BUD: Yes.

BOYNE: Do they live nearby?

BUD: Yes.

BOYNE: Do you see them regularly?

BUD: No.

BOYNE: Do you visit them?

BUD: No.

BOYNE: Do they visit you?

BUD: They did one time, but not anymore.

BOYNE: Do you have a good relationship with them, or not so good, or terrible?

BUD: I don't have a good relationship with them at all.

BOYNE: Do they visit their mother?

BUD: Yes.

BOYNE: Does she visit them?

BUD: I assume she does.

BOYNE: Do you think she has a better relationship with them than you have?

BUD: Oh, I'm sure she does.

BOYNE: You said you spent thirty-five years working and buying the home and keeping a roof over their head. How do you feel about the way it's all turned out?

BUD: Well, I don't like it. I didn't want it that way. All my life I wanted a wife and children, a family, a home, but it didn't work out that way.

BOYNE: How long have you been divorced?

BUD: I'd say thirty-four years now.

BOYNE: Thirty-four years divorced. How long did your marriage last?

BUD: About three years.

BOYNE: What is it that kept you from remarrying?

BUD: I had my opportunities, but I had to take care of my mother and dad until he died, and now I still have my mother.

BOYNE: So the word alcoholic is objectionable to you. From your point of view, that label doesn't fit you.

BUD: I don't believe it does, no.

BOYNE: How does alcohol benefit you? First let me find the setting. Is all or most of your drinking done as solitary drinking or is all or most of your drinking done in other settings—barrooms, clubs, social clubs, card clubs, and so on?

BUD: No, I drink alone in my house.

BOYNE: You're a solitary drinker?

BUD: Yes. I have a lady friend, and when we go to eat, we have a couple of drinks before and a couple afterwards. I take her home and that's the evening. But otherwise when I get down to serious drinking, as I call it, I do it in the privacy of my own home.

BOYNE: How do you benefit from the alcohol? What does alcohol do for you at this point?

BUD: Well, it relaxes me for one thing, and when I'm drinking brandy, it seems like I can think better. You know, things are more clear to me.

BOYNE: Suppose I said that while you are drinking, you're not thinking those same critical, self-condemning thoughts about yourself.

BUD: No, I'm not. It seems like if I have any problems when I'm drinking brandy, I can seem to iron them out; but then again the whole next day it's all different.

BOYNE: Remember W. C. Fields?

BUD: Yes, I do (laughter).

BOYNE: He believed that his comedic genius could only be released with alcohol, and it was true. He always did have a jug of martinis on the set. Remember John Barrymore?

BUD: Yes, sure do.

BOYNE: John was considered by many to be in his early years one of the greatest classical actors of our time. But he came to believe that he could only release his talent through alcohol and become a travesty of himself.

BUD: Yes.

BOYNE: Remember Edgar Allen Poe?

BUD: I read his works.

BOYNE: He reached a point where he believed that he could only release his writing talent through alcohol. You see, many people develop a belief that they need a drink or two to steady their nerves.

BUD: (He nods in agreement.)

BOYNE: I had an uncle like that. Last time I saw him he got so steady he didn't move for three days.

BUD: (Laughter)

BOYNE: Now here's the rule. First the thought, then the action, then the habit of thinking and the habit of acting, then the compulsive thinking and the compulsive action. So if you believe that the only way you can be free of these feelings that have plagued you all those years is with brandy, and then you act upon it by drinking the brandy, and then you do it again, and over and over again, you're into compulsive behavior, aren't you? Compulsive means you don't have control over it.

BUD: Oh, I believe that I do have control. I don't believe I'm an alcoholic.

BOYNE: Not a falling down one anyway.

BUD: No, sir, I'm not. (Laughter as Gil clasps Bud's arm.)

BOYNE: So the word alcoholic is a pretty tough word for you to accept.

BUD: No, I'm not alcoholic.

BOYNE: Okay. You just drink a lot.

BUD: At times.

BOYNE: You said, "I don't feel anything." How about when you've had your eight ounces of brandy, do your feelings seem a little more open? Do you ever sit down and watch the late, late movie and when there's a sentimental scene maybe cry a few tears?

BUD: Well, I don't need brandy to get emotional about a sentimental movie. I guess I am an emotional person.

Really. I have it worse than some women.

BOYNE: Tell me about that.

BUD: I don't really know what to say except at the movies, at a sad movie, it always seems somehow I can relate to it and it bothers me.

BOYNE: I hear you saying, you're very aware of a sadness within you.

BUD: Well, I'm not a happy man.

BOYNE: I hear you saying that there is a great longing within you that never gets satisfied.

BUD: That's true because I'm not living a life that I want to live. I'm not free to live the life I'd like to live.

BOYNE: How old is your mother?

BUD: She's eighty-three.

BOYNE: And the state of her health?

BUD: She's good physically; mentally, not so good.

BOYNE: You've been here now a day and a half observing and listening as we talk about and demonstrate some of the processes of hypnosis as a tool for reaching the deeper mind and the feeling level. Give me a brief readout of your thoughts and feelings about what's been happening.

BUD: Well, I'm not so sure exactly. This is another thing that bothers me—that all of you people are educated and I'm not. I can't express myself like the rest of you.

BOYNE: Can you go into a diner and order ham and eggs?

BUD: Sure.

BOYNE: Then you have the power to communicate, don't you? What are your thoughts and feelings about what's been going on?

BUD: Well, all the time I'm watching what's been going on

here, I've been thinking I wish you could do for me what you've done for these people. That's what I want.

BOYNE: Did you identify with any of the people, the case histories that you've seen? Could you connect with them at a feeling level?

BUD: Well, this morning when John grabbed your arm there and screamed at you, I almost came out of my chair because I thought that was a very emotional thing.

BOYNE: That was probably the least emotional thing that we did.

BUD: Is that right?

BOYNE: It might have been the loudest.

BUD: But I thought it was emotional. I almost put myself in his shoes.

BOYNE: Have you ever been hypnotized?

BUD: Never.

BOYNE: Previous to coming here, have you ever seen anyone hypnotized?

BUD: No, sir.

BOYNE: Not even in a nightclub or on television or in a show of any kind?

BUD: I may have on television.

BOYNE: Now that you've been here and seen a few people hypnotized, is hypnosis as you believed or imagined it might be?

BUD: I think so, yes.

BOYNE: Is it in any way different from what you thought it would be?

BUD: Oh, when you get forceful, I never figured on that, but then that's your way of doing things. No, I thought you just talked to the subject, he answers, you ask him questions, he answers you; and I guess that's pretty much what you've been doing.

BOYNE: You said you didn't know therapists get forceful. What does that refer to?

BUD: I thought you got a little bit rough with that girl, Jackie, and the same with John here. You had him screaming. You know, you were hollering at him and he was hollering back at you. I didn't expect anything like that.

BOYNE: So it surprised you.

BUD: Yes.

BOYNE: I suspect it would surprise most that don't know very much about it. Are you ready for me to hypnotize you?

BUD: Yes, sir, I am.

BOYNE: Now you can stand. Turn and face me if you will. Take a step forward. Now pull your feet together in close. SLEEP! (Gil pulls Bud's head forward.) Turn loose now. Relax. Let a good, pleasant feeling now come all across your body. Let each muscle and nerve grow loose and limp and relaxed. Turn all the neck muscles loose. That's good. Breathing easily and deeply, (Gil rotates Bud's head as says) and relaxing more with each easy breath that you take. Your arms grow limp, just like a rag doll. (Gil picks up Bud's arms and lets them drop to his sides.) You're feeling more and more relaxed with each passing second. Turning loose and letting go. Calmly, quietly, easily, and gently.

Listen carefully now. (Gil supports Bud's neck with one arm and his other hand is on Bud's forehead.) I'm going to count from five down to one, and as I do, you're eyelids lock so tightly closed, the more you try to open them, the tighter they're locking closed. Five, eyelids pressing down tightly. Four, they're pressing down and sealing shut. Three, they're sealing as if they were glued. Two, they're locked. The more you try to open them now, the tighter they're locking closed. One, try to open them and see they're stuck tight. You can stop trying. Relax and just sleep deeply. (Gil snaps his fingers and moves Bud's head forward.) Head forward onto your chest, and you go much deeper. That's good. Down and deeper. Arms limp, loosely, limply relaxing. Now I'm going to turn your body a little bit. I want you to take a step forward with your left foot. That's it. Then pull back and come right into this chair. I'm going to press you down now so that you can sit down into the chair. That's it.

Now you're into the chair, and you can sit comfortably and as you do, you continue relaxing. I want you now to focus your awareness down to your right hand. I'm going to count from one up to twenty, and as I do a light, easy, pleasant feeling moves into your right hand and into your arm. As I continue counting that feeling grows stronger and stronger. Soon you will feel the first slight movement, slight movement of the fingers and twitching of the muscles. Then your hand begins to lighten, your arm begins to lift, and it continues moving and lifting and rising until it comes to rest over on your body or maybe up on your chest or even on your chin or up on your cheek. (Gil takes Bud's hand and demonstrates the movement for Bud.) When you feel that movement in your hand and in your arm, don't try to resist. You could resist if you chose to, that's not why you're here. Let your subconscious mind do its perfect work.

Now we begin. Focus your attention now down to your right hand and without moving your fingers become aware of the material of your trousers beneath your finger tips. Focus your attention right into the pulse beating in your wrist (Gil touches Bud's wrist) and see if you can pick up an awareness of that pulse. That's going to take a little fine tuning on your part. As I count from one up to twenty, that light, easy, pleasant feeling moves into your right hand and quickly it begins to move and to lift and to rise and to float. Number one, the first light, easy sensation moves into the finger tips of your right hand. Number two, the feeling is spreading around beneath the finger-nails. On number three, it's moving up to the first joint of the finger. Number four, spreading through the large knuckle across the back of the hand. Number five, soon the first slight movements begin taking place, slight movements of the fingers, a twitching of the muscles. That's good. On number six, the light sensation continues spreading as it's moving across the back of the hand. Number eight, spreading over and into your thumb from the finger tips all the way up across the back of the hand, over and into your thumb. Your right hand has grown light and free and it's ready to lift.

Number nine, think of your left hand now and you'll see it's beginning to feel as heavy as lead. Your left hand is feeling so heavy now while on number ten, your right hand grows lighter, lighter with each number I count, as light as a feather floating in the breeze and even lighter, as light as a gas filled balloon. Just as a gas filled balloon will rise and float toward the ceiling, in the same way by the time I reach the count of twenty (Bud's hand begins to twitch), your right hand is moving, and lifting and rising and floating. Eleven, the light sensation is into the wrist and beyond. From the finger tips up to the wrist and beyond, your right hand is light and free and lifting. On number twelve, your left hand feels as heavy as lead. While on thirteen your right hand is moving, lifting, rising. Thirteen, as you feel those movements now, just let it continue moving, lifting, and rising. That's good. You've got the knack of it now. Just let it continue as your hand is moving and lifting and rising, coming up and moving up until it comes up to rest upon your body.

Now the instant your hand touches your body, you'll become more relaxed than you've been in a very long time. Fourteen, that light sensation moves right on up toward your elbow. Fifteen, your hand is moving in and coming up, moving and lifting and rising, coming in and moving up. On number fifteen, into the elbow from the finger tips all the way up to the elbow, your hand is light and free and lifting. Just as light as a feather floating in the breeze and even lighter, as light as a gas filled balloon. Just as that gas filled balloon will rise and float toward the ceiling, by the time I reach the count of twenty, your right hand is up on your body; and when it touches your body, you'll feel yourself drifting to a much deeper level of relaxation and slumber.

Sixteen, as your hand is free and lifting, you're relaxing more than ever before. Seventeen, coming up and moving up now, all the way up until it comes to rest upon your body. Eighteen, as your hand is lifting, you're going deeper and deeper into hypnosis. Nineteen, your left arm feels as though it were made of marble or stone or lead. When your hand touches your body, your left arm feels so heavy that just the very thought of lifting it is more than you want to concern yourself with. (Bud is moving his right hand toward his body.) The right hand is coming up on nineteen, and now it's about to come to rest upon your body. Number twenty, your hand is coming to rest upon your body and at the same time your left hand has grown so heavy, it feels as though it were made of marble or stone or lead—you may if you wish make an effort to lift your left arm, but you'll find it's more than you want to concern yourself with now. It feels as though it were impossible for you to lift.

This time I'll tap your forehead. As I do, your right hand drops down, and you go much deeper into hypnosis. Drop it down and go deeper. (Gil taps Bud's forehead.) That's fine. There's a feeling about yourself. It's a feeling that you can't do anything right. It's a feeling of being criticized, a feeling of being unloved. It's a feeling of being unlovable. It's a feeling that causes you to feel nervous, tense, anxious, fearful, frightened, afraid. As I count from one up to ten, I want you to become aware of that feeling. One, two, three, now the feeling begins to emerge. Four, five, it's a feeling that you're just a klutz, you never do anything right. Six, you're bound to be thought dumb and stupid. Seven, no one loves you. Eight, you're all alone. Nine, it's like the floodgates on a dam opening up and a great wave of feeling is rolling across you now. Number ten, this time I'll count to three and tap your forehead. I'm going to ask you a question. The answer will come out by spelling letter by letter. One, two, three. (Gil taps Bud's forehead as he counts.) What is it that causes you to feel tense, nervous, anxious, fearful, afraid? The first letter, quickly. Speak out.

BUD: F.

BOYNE: The next.

BUD: Fear.

BOYNE: I'm going to tap your forehead again. You'll speak a sentence, a phrase, or a paragraph that incorporates the word *fear*. Speak.

BUD: I'm afraid to say anything for fear that I'm going to be wrong or make a mistake.

BOYNE: All right. Now I'm going to count from ten down to one. As I do, we're going to an earlier time that has to do with this same feeling of fear. Ten, nine, eight, we're drifting back. Seven, six, five, you're growing younger now. Four, your arms and legs are shrinking and you're growing smaller. Three, two, one. (Gil taps Bud's forehead.) Where are you now? Are you indoors or outside? Make a choice quickly. Pick one.

BUD: I'm outdoors.

BOYNE: Daytime or nighttime?

BUD: Daytime.

BOYNE: You're outdoors, it's in the daytime. Are you alone or is someone with you?

BUD: Someone is with me.

BOYNE: Who is it that's with you?

BUD: A schoolmate.

BOYNE: You're with your schoolmates. How old are you?

BUD: Five or six.

BOYNE: What's going on? Give a report.

BUD: We're fighting.

BOYNE: Fighting in the schoolyard?

BUD: Yes, sir.

BOYNE: Are just you and one other boy fighting, or a group fighting?

BUD: Just the other boy and I.

BOYNE: How do you feel about the fight? Are you afraid of him or do you think you can whip him?

BUD: Well, I'm afraid of him as he is of me.

BOYNE: You're both afraid. That's the way it usually is. What's happening now?

BUD: I'm chasing him home.

BOYNE: He's running away from you?

BUD: Yes, sir.

BOYNE: How do you feel?

BUD: Feel all right.

BOYNE: Go ahead a little bit in time now and tell me what you're experiencing. Have you arrived home yet?

BUD: Yes, sir.

BOYNE: And does your mother or anyone at home know about this fight yet?

BUD: My dad.

BOYNE: Your dad. All right. When I tap your forehead, you're with your dad. It's about the fight.

BUD: I tell him about the fight. He wants to know more about it. I tell him, "One night I chase him home, the next night he chases me home."

BOYNE: What does Dad say to that?

BUD: He says, "The next time he chases you home, I'm going to give you a licking when you get here."

BOYNE: The next time that you show that you're afraid, then you're going to really have to be afraid because your father is going to give you a licking for being afraid; is that right?

BUD: That's right.

BOYNE: I'll count from one to four and when I do, you go to another time that has to do with this fear. One, two, three, four. (Gil taps Bud's forehead.) Are you indoors or outside?

BUD: I'm outside.

BOYNE: Daytime or nighttime?

BUD: Daytime.

BOYNE: Are you alone or is someone with you?

BUD: Someone is with me.

BOYNE: Who is it that's with you?

BUD: Another schoolmate.

BOYNE: You're with your schoolmate. How old are you?

BUD: Probably sixteen.

BOYNE: You're sixteen years old. What's going on?

BUD: We're having a fight.

BOYNE: How do you feel?

BUD: Not too good.

BOYNE: What's happening?

BUD: I have a carbuncle on my neck and the guy's got his arm around my neck squeezing on me.

BOYNE: I bet that really hurts, doesn't it?

BUD: Yes, sir.

BOYNE: He's squeezing where your carbuncle is on the neck?

BUD: That's right.

BOYNE: Is he asking you to give up or give in?

BUD: I told him I had to give in, I had enough.

BOYNE: All right. Is there anyone around watching?

BUD: Yes, sir.

BOYNE: How do you feel?

BUD: I'm not very happy about it because nobody knows about the carbuncle except my close friend.

BOYNE: What do you think that those watching the fight are thinking about you?

BUD: That I'm a coward.

BOYNE: That you're a coward; that you're full of fear. When I count to four, we'll go to one more experience that has to do with this same feeling. One, two, three, four.

(Gil snaps his fingers at each count and then taps Bud's forehead.) Once again, are you indoors or outside?

BUD: I'm outside.

BOYNE: Is it daytime or nighttime?

BUD: It's nighttime.

BOYNE: Are you alone or is someone with you?

BUD: Someone's with me.

BOYNE: Who is it that's with you?

BUD: An army buddy.

BOYNE: You're with your army buddy. How old are you?

BUD: Twenty-one.

BOYNE: Twenty-one. What's happening?

BUD: We're at a boxing bout, and when I go to stand up, somebody throws a rock, hits me in the head. So I go over and punch him.

BOYNE: Now you've hit him with your fists. What's happening?

BUD: Well, I hit him three or four times and that's the end of it. Somebody's standing there saying, "We've got a better one going on here than they got in the ring."

BOYNE: How do you feel about that?

BUD: I don't like to fight.

BOYNE: What is the inner feeling when you fight?

BUD: I'm disgusted with myself.

BOYNE: Disgusted that your anger and frustration and rage broke loose.

BUD: Yes, sir.

BOYNE: All right. (Gil rests his hand on Bud's forehead as he is says) Let your mind grow clear. I'll count from one up to ten. Come up to this time, 1985. One, two, three, four, five, six, seven, eight, nine, ten. The month of April, city of Chicago, 1985. I want you to listen carefully. I'm going to have you go back and look at this with your adult mind and analyze the experiences of the boy and his fear and how his father locked him into a cycle of fear and so on. Understand how it affected his thinking and how it affected his behavior as he grew and how it may even be affecting you today. When you've done that, and you're ready to talk about it, just raise your hand like this (Gil raises Bud's hand in demonstration), and we'll talk about it then. All right. Three, two, one. (Gil is tapping Bud's forehead.) Now look back and examine the experiences of the young boy.

BUD: I just don't know what to say. I—at no time in my life did I ever want to fight, but it seemed like I was always fighting. I wasn't very good, but sometimes I got pretty lucky. I wish that I could have talked my way out of it, but I was never a very good talker, and I haven't changed my mind to this day.

BOYNE: Haven't changed your mind about?

BUD: Fighting. I hate it. I hate it with a passion, and when I see other people fight, I'm disgusted with them.

BOYNE: In a moment I'm going to have you open your eyes. Before I do, is there anything further you want to say to me, ask me, or tell me in this session?

BUD: I can't think of anything.

BOYNE: All right. (Gil taps Bud's arm and says) Quickly now, who do I remind you of?

BUD: Tommy Lasorda.

BOYNE: How do I remind you of Tommy Lasorda?

BUD: Well, you look like him.

BOYNE: Any qualities you feel I share with Tommy Lasorda?

BUD: You're both good men.

BOYNE: When I count from one up to five, let your eyelids open, you're calm, rested, refreshed, relaxed. You feel good. One, slowly, calmly, easily, and gently returning to your full awareness once again. Two, each muscle and nerve in your body is loose and limp and relaxed, and you feel good. Three, from head to toe you're feeling perfect in every way. On number four, your eyes begin to feel sparkling clear. On the next number now, eyelids open, fully aware, feeling wonderfully good. Number five, eyelids open, look right over here at me. (Gil and Bud laugh.) Well, you kind of surprised yourself, didn't you?

BUD: I sure did.

BOYNE: Tell me about it.

BUD: (He dries his eyes.) Okay. I almost got carried away there when you asked me to go back in time.

BOYNE: You did very good work.

BUD: Thank you.

BOYNE: What are your thoughts about all this that went on?

BUD: Well, I'm just tickled to death I had it done. I just hope it all works out for me.

BOYNE: We'll do some more work on you tomorrow. Can you come back tomorrow?

BUD: Yes, sir, I can. Be happy to come back.

BOYNE: You're going to have some wonderful dreams tonight. They're going to start preparing you for a gigantic breakthrough tomorrow.

BUD: Good.

BOYNE: Is that agreeable to you?

BUD: Oh, it certainly is. I'm very happy about it.

BOYNE: (Gil faces the class to speak.) This was a very typical first session illustrating that all problems are really problems of fear and there are only a few basic fears. The fears are: the fear of criticism; the fear of rejection, which is the feeling of being unloved; a fear of sickness and aging; fear of death; fear of poverty and not being in control of one's finances. When we focus upon those and deal with them in a creative way, we can discover the way that our energy has been mobilized and then paralyzed to maintain frustrating behavior patterns.

Until the next time, this is Gil Boyne.

THE CASE OF BUD
"Born to Lose"
Session Two

(The Setting: A Hypnotherapy Class in Chicago)

(BOYNE ADDRESSES THE AUDIENCE)

BOYNE: Hello. This is Gil Boyne, and welcome back to our Hypnotherapy Video Clinic. Today we're back with Bud for session number two.

(BOYNE ADDRESSES BUD)

Bud, it's been about twenty-four hours since we worked together here. Tell me about your thoughts and feelings since the work we did yesterday.

BUD: Well, when I went home last night to the hotel, I had the best sleep I've had in several months.

BOYNE: Wonderful.

BUD: Yes. I went to bed about ten o'clock, and I woke up at five o'clock this morning just wide awake.

BOYNE: You logged seven hours of good sound sleep.

BUD: And I didn't need any five-star brandy to do it. I didn't need any help.

BOYNE: Wasn't that a good feeling?

BUD: It certainly was, and I feel more relaxed. I'm a little apprehensive today, nervous, but I guess it's normal. But I feel a lot better than I did yesterday when I came in.

BOYNE: Were you aware of any dream activity during the night?

BUD: No.

BOYNE: Just a good sound sleep.

BUD: That's right.

BOYNE: That's a fine report about your sleeping. What are your thoughts about some of the things that you re-called and remembered, things we talked about here yesterday, things that related to your past and to your present?

BUD: Well, they're things I hadn't thought of in all these years, you know, I had completely forgot about them. I am surprised that these things came up, that I was able to think of these certain points.

BOYNE: Your subconscious selected those incidents to illus-trate certain fears within you.

BUD: Yes.

BOYNE: What was it that you uncovered? What did you learn from that session?

BUD: Well, I'm a great one for always looking back, but last night I couldn't make myself go back in the past and think about all the things that I've done wrong or the bad things that's happened to me. I couldn't think of anything in the past.

(BOYNE ADDRESSES THE AUDIENCE)

BOYNE: "To think of all the things that I've done wrong." Many people are insomniacs because they get into bed and they review the day, and they're not reviewing what they did that was appropriate or successful. They're looking upon their mistakes or the things they might have done better, which is the perfection-ist: "I could have done that a little better. Why did I tell that joke to Fred at lunch time about the Catholic priest? I should have remembered his brother was a priest. I'm so stupid," and on and on. And then the real insomniacs, once they get past the day, they go back into the week and then having remembered all their mistakes of the week. They go back into the month and the year, and pretty soon they're remem-bering that time when they were twelve years old and they were at a concert and heard the nphony orchestra for the very first time, and in een movements they applauded and everyone turi nd looked at them.

(BOYNE ADDRESSES BUD)

All the while they keep running the tip of tongue around inside their mouth to see if they c nd any new cavities. That's called catastrophic ex itions. "If I look for trouble hard enough, I'll fin ' You said, "As I thought back over all the thi did wrong." Those who suffer from an intens r of criticism are critical of others, but most intens itical of themselves, and that's what you just saic

Please continue.

BUD: Well, my mind just blanked out everything in th
Normally I can go back twenty years thinking of t
maybe I should have done differently, should
said differently. I could have saved myself a lot of
times, so to speak.

BOYNE: That's a form of silliness called "regrets."

BUD: It's true. That's right.

BOYNE: One of your favorite exercises, isn't it?

BUD: It sure is and it's cost me a lot of sleepless nights.

(BOYNE ADDRESSES THE AUDIENCE)

BOYNE: You begin to see some of the causes in those people who say, "I just can't sleep at night." It is natural to sleep. Every organism has a dormant period which is regular and cyclical. It's unnatural to stay awake when you've been up for a sufficient period of time.

BUD: (He sighs.)

BOYNE: Insomnia is always brought about by something that the person is doing mentally. You are now hearing some of the things that they do. Please continue.

BUD: Well, it's because I've always gone back and thought about these things, how I would do them differently. I've got to where I would go to bed, and I would lay there night after night, and this went on for a good many months. I'd get up disgusted and I'd go drink some brandy to make me sleepy, and then go back to bed when I felt sleepy. Then I'd get up with two or three hours sleep, and this went on time and again. After last night, I felt completely rested this morning.

BOYNE: So the first thing that's happening to you now is that you know it's not impossible or it's not even difficult for you to go to sleep without brandy.

BUD: That's right.

BOYNE: You didn't know that until last night. How much is that information worth to you?

BUD: An awful lot.

BOYNE: Wasn't it yesterday you remembered about fighting?

BUD: Well, school days. First, trouble I get into fighting with one of the kids.

BOYNE: Tell me about your thoughts about the fighting. You said that you got into a lot of fights, but then you felt disgusted afterwards.

BUD: I just don't like it, but I would do it because my dad told me one time, (Gil draws closer and becomes more intent as Bud is talking) he said, "If you run home again, then I'll give you a licking, so you better not come running home." And I never did again. I had a lot of fights. But I never liked it—I always thought that it was something I had to do, that it was the manly thing to do.

BOYNE: Say that again.

BUD: As I grew older, I thought it was the manly thing to do.

BOYNE: Turn the sentence around and say, "As I grew older, I was afraid of being called a coward."

BUD: As I grew older, I was afraid of being called a coward, and in this town where I came from, if you turned away you were called a coward.

BOYNE: Then you were in real trouble, weren't you?

BUD: Yes, I was.

BOYNE: They'd beat up on you every day.

BUD: Well, they'd kick your butt every time you showed your face outside.

BOYNE: I want to tell you, I was a fighter for a gang that I belonged to in the ghetto. Back then it was innocent fighting. We fought with our fists and we didn't use zip guns or weapons. I remember I fought one man, a fighter for another gang, thirty-seven times. Sometimes I'd win, sometimes he'd win; but I never enjoyed it and I never looked forward to it.

BUD: No.

BOYNE: And I never thought that it was a good thing to do but I knew I had to do it.

BUD: (He nods in agreement.)

BOYNE: Because every time we would meet, one of us would say, "Knock that off my shoulder." You know what that meant.

BUD: Sure.

BOYNE: If you turned and walked away, what happened?

BUD: You were called "chicken."

BOYNE: You were in serious trouble, weren't you?

BUD: You sure were.

BOYNE: So I understand that feeling. We can become addicted to pumping of the adrenaline. The proof of it is that they can make a motion picture showing an actor like Clint Eastwood as a man who travels the country streetfighting with his bare knuckles at industrial plants and behind dirty barrooms. He is a great folk hero because he always manages to win even though he may get cut up and scarred. I had an uncle who was a barroom fighter, Uncle Joe. He lost an eye in one fight and three years later he was killed on a barroom floor. It makes me wonder why motion pictures like that roll up big box office grosses. There seems to be something glamorous about fist fighting with the real tough guys. It is one of the most stupid things I've ever seen.

BUD: That's right, but that's what people like to see.

BOYNE: At least certain kinds of people do. And both of us were once that kind of person. Interesting how there's such an opportunity to market such insane values to the Saturday-night-movie crowd. The people who write those films would rather exploit certain brutal aspects of human nature than to make a contribution to the development of human values.

BUD: More money in it, I suppose.

BOYNE: So you fought a lot and never really liked it, but you didn't want to be labeled a coward and your father said, "By God, if you show the white feather, you're in trouble with me."

BUD: That's right.

BOYNE: One day I came running into the house and my father said, "What's going on?" I said, "There's three of them chasing me." He said, "You go out the front and walk down the street; I'm going out the back alley and we'll see what happens." So I did and just about the time I hit the corner, they jumped me and he grabbed two of them. He prided himself on being a tough guy, and he just said to them, "You fight him one at a time." So I fought one and then when he gave up, I had to fight the other one. I won both fights only because I was afraid not to. If you were to ask me, "Did anything positive come out of that?" I would answer yes. I learned that it's not being tough, it's knowing you can win despite the fear. It's knowing the other guy has fear too, and knowing that you have to do battle. I'm now characterizing a difference between you and me. I'm a winner and I've been a winner much of my life. You told us you're a loser.

BUD: I told you that, yes.

BOYNE: Isn't it interesting that we have such similar backgrounds!

BUD: Yes.

BOYNE: That's called inferiority feelings versus goal strivings. In other words, how the inferiority feelings are created in our early developmental stages and how we deal with them. Some of us become overcompensators and some become undercompensators.

BUD: (He nods in agreement.)

BOYNE: There are problems in overachievement, and overcompensating, but there are also great rewards. There are a damned few rewards in undercompensation.

BUD: That's right, I know. (Gil and Bud shake hands.)

BOYNE: I think we're talking the same language. You're eyes are moist. Can you tell me what's going on?

BUD: I don't know.

BOYNE: Close your eyes. Go into yourself. Become aware of your feelings. What are you experiencing?

BUD: I think I'm peaceful and relaxed.

BOYNE: Open our eyes. Now turn your head and look at me. I'm going to count from five down to one, as I do you're eyes grow heavy, droopy, drowsy, and sleepy.

By the time I reach the count of one, they close right down and go deep into hypnotic slumber. Five, eyelids heavy, droopy, drowsy, and sleepy. Four, the next time they blink, that's hypnosis coming on you then. Three, your heavy lids are ready to close. Two, they begin closing, closing, closing, closing, close them, close them, close them. (Gil moves Bud's head forward at same time he says) One, SLEEP! Turn loose now. Relax. Let a good, pleasant feeling come all across your body. That's it. Let each muscle and nerve begin to grow loose and limp and relaxed. Let your arms grow limp now, just like a rag doll. (Gil picks up Bud's left hand by Bud's thumb.) So when I drop them, let them drop just like a rag dropping to the floor. That's it. Loosely, limply, relaxing way down. Now you've got it. There's a feeling about yourself. It's a feeling that has to do with feeling fearful, nervous, anxious. It's that kind of feeling that has to do with fighting, feeling disgusted about it. As I count from one up to ten, I want you to become aware of that feeling. One, two, three, it's that feeling of disgust. Four, five, six, it's that feeling of fear. Seven, eight, the fear of anger. Nine, ten, it causes you to be tense, nervous, fearful, anxious. When I count to three once again, I'll tap your forehead and ask you a question. One, two, three. What is it now that causes you to have these kinds of feelings?

BUD: Insecurity.

BOYNE: Insecurity. That's a vague and general term. I want you to give me a more specific word. What is it that causes you to feel nervous and tense and anxious and fearful and frightened so much of the time? Tell me now.

BUD: I'm just not sure of myself.

BOYNE: I didn't ask what you're sure of. Give me an answer.

BUD: I don't—guess I'm just afraid of being made a fool of.

BOYNE: And you've made a fool of yourself all of your life, haven't you?

BUD: Yes, sir.

BOYNE: I'm going to count from ten down to one. Let's go to an earlier time that has to do with this same kind of feeling. Ten, nine, eight, drifting back. Seven, six, five, growing younger now. Four, your arms and legs are shrinking, you're growing smaller. Three, two, one. Where you are now, are you indoors or outside?

BUD: Outside.

BOYNE: Daytime or nighttime?

BUD: Daytime.

BOYNE: Are you alone or is someone with you?

BUD: Someone's with me.

BOYNE: Who is it that's with you?

BUD: Playmate.

BOYNE: How old are you?

BUD: About six.

BOYNE: Six years old. What's going on?

BUD: I have a bag of candy and I'm showing my friend the candy. It's in the summertime, and he puts his hand in the bag and grabs a whole handful of candy, and I hit him. He goes crying to his dad, and my dad told me to come over and sit on the porch and stay there until he told me I could go. After awhile my friend came out. He said, "Come on over and play." I went over, we were playing. My dad cut a willow stick off of a willow tree, and he came and got me and he started beating me with that stick. I was naked from the waist up and from the knees down, and he laced me pretty good with that stick. I remember my mother telling him to stop it or she would call the police.

BOYNE: Now be there, hear your mother screaming. What's happening?

BUD: He stopped beating me.

BOYNE: Let your mind grow clear. (Gil places his hand on Bud's forehead and then places his hand on the back of Bud's neck.) This time when I count to three, your father is seated in the chair about eight feet out in front of you, and you're seated in the chair facing him. One, two, three. There sits your father. I want you to talk to him now. How would you address him? Do you call him Dad, Pop, Poppa?

BUD: I call him Dad.

BOYNE: Say, "Dad, I want to talk to you."

BUD: Dad, I want to talk to you.

BOYNE: "I want to tell you my feelings."

BUD: I want to tell you my feelings.

BOYNE: Now tell him.

BUD: There's times when I hate you.

BOYNE: Say it again.

BUD: There are times when I hate you.

BOYNE: Again. What's happening?

BUD: There are times when I hate you.

BOYNE: Listen to me. Look over to your dad and say, "I hate your guts."

BUD: I hate your guts.

BOYNE: Say it LOUDER!

BUD: I hate your guts.

BOYNE: LOUDER!

BUD: I hate your guts.

BOYNE: LOUDER!

BUD: I hate your guts.

BOYNE: SCREAM IT!

BUD: I HATE YOUR GUTS!

BOYNE: Again.

BUD: I HATE YOUR GUTS!

BOYNE: Once again.

BUD: I HATE YOU!

BOYNE: Again.

BUD: I HATE YOU! (He waves his arms as he screams.)

BOYNE: All right. Rest. I want you now to change places. Be the father. Answer your son. Speak to your son who says that he hates you.

BUD: (As the father) Why do you hate me?

BOYNE: Be the son. Father wants to know why you hate him.

BUD: Because you gave me this terrible licking. When I ask you something, you never answer me. If you do, it's always "mallet head, blockhead, or dummy." You never spend any time with me. I heard my mother say to you one time that you didn't want me. We were in a garden, it was in the summertime, I was hauling trash out in the rear of the garden, you denied it. I heard what you said.

BOYNE: Be the father. Answer your son.

BUD: (As the father) This is not true. This is not true.

BOYNE: Be the boy.

BUD: But I know it is. I heard you say it. I heard my mother say it. She wouldn't lie.

BOYNE: Be the father.

BUD: (As the father) I never, I never said it. I didn't mean it if I did.

BOYNE: Say that again.

BUD: (As the father) I didn't mean it if I did.

BOYNE: Again.

BUD: (As the father) I never meant it if I did.

BOYNE: Do you love your son?

BUD: (As the father) Yeah, I love the boy.

BOYNE: Tell him that.

BUD: (As the father) Yes, I do.

BOYNE: Tell your son you love him.

BUD: (As the father) Son, I love you.

BOYNE: You know sometimes we have difficulty expressing love because of the way our parents treated us. Maybe you can explain to your son some of your problems in not being able to make him feel loved. Talk to him now. How do you call your son? What's his name?

BUD: (As the father) Bud.

BOYNE: Call him.

BUD: (As the father) Bud, let me talk to you. If I've done you wrong, I want to make it up to you. We can do things together. We can go fishing. We can go to ball games.

BOYNE: Tell him how it was with your parents. (Bud leans forward to hear the statement again.) Tell him how it was with your father, the way he behaved toward you.

BUD: (As the father) My dad didn't take me to ball games. Once in awhile he would take me fishing. He just never would sit down and talk to me.

BOYNE: Be the boy.

BUD: (He sighs deeply.) I just, I don't know what to say. I just—

BOYNE: Say, "Why don't you ever compliment me? Why don't you ever praise me? Why don't you ever say something to make me feel good?" Ask him that.

BUD: Dad, why don't you ever compliment me? Why don't you ever praise me? Why don't you ever say anything that makes me feel good?

BOYNE: Be the father. Answer that.

BUD: (As the father) I don't know, son. I guess I take you for granted. I don't know.

BOYNE: Be the boy. Answer your father.

BUD: But I need to hear this. I don't know half the time whether I'm right or wrong. If I'm doing wrong, I want to know. If I'm doing right, I want to know that too.

BOYNE: Be the father.

BUD: (As the father) From now on, son, I'll try and do these things for you. When you do something right, I'll tell you. When you're doing something wrong, you're going to know that too.

BOYNE: (Gil puts his hand on Bud's forehead and says) Let your mind grow clear. Your father sits out there in the chair. I want you to repeat after me. "I'm not put in this world to live up to what you expect of me."

BUD: I'm not put in this world to live up to what you expect of me.

BOYNE: Tell him what it means.

BUD: No love.

BOYNE: Now say this. "You're not put in this world to live up to what I have expected of you."

BUD: You're not put in this world to live up to what I expect of you.

BOYNE: Tell him what that means.

BUD: I don't know what it means. I just—

BOYNE: That's where you're stuck. Because you can never escape those critical demands of that parent figure so long as you feel that you have to get something from that person. I'm proposing that the reason you felt unloved all these years is that you're stuck waiting for your father to change, waiting for your father to love you, waiting for that emptiness to be filled, and you've become a bottomless pit. You can't be nourished by what others give you. You won't recognize love. You don't recognize love when it surrounds you. It doesn't nourish you. You're still stuck back there. Come up to this time and place as I count from one up to ten. One, two, three, four, five, six, seven, eight, nine, ten. (Gil places his hand on Bud's forehead as he counts.) This is 1985. You're growing older now. I want you to listen very carefully now. This is 1985 and you're a grown man, sixty-one, is that correct?

BUD: That's right.

BOYNE: Is your father alive or deceased?

BUD: He's dead.

BOYNE: Where were you when your father died?

BUD: I was working on my job.

BOYNE: Living at home?

BUD: I was living at the YMCA.

BOYNE: How did you learn of your father's death?

BUD: They called the place where I was working.

BOYNE: Tell me your first feeling?

BUD: I really didn't have much feeling. I just expected it.

BOYNE: How old were you when your father died?

BUD: (He sighs deeply.) I would say forty-seven.

SAYING "GOOD-BYE"

BOYNE: Forty-seven. When I count to three, you're going to

be in the room, your father's in the bed, he's dying, but I'm going to give you a chance to talk to him. (As Gil counts to three, he taps Bud's forehead.) One, two, three. Now you're sitting in a chair along side the bed. There's your father. He's going to die in a very short time. I want you to talk to him and say, "Dad, before you go, there's some things I want to say to you." Begin.

BUD: Dad, before you go, there's some things I'd like to say to you.

BOYNE: Speak to him now.

BUD: After all these years, I would like to know how you really felt about me.

BOYNE: Be the father. Your son wants to know how you really felt about him.

BUD: (As the father) Son, I never hated you. I know I probably wasn't the best father. I know I was temperamental. Maybe that's why I didn't show affection like I should have. I'm just incapable of doing it.

BOYNE: Say that again.

BUD: (As the father) I was not capable of showing affection.

BOYNE: Say, "I did the best I could even if it wasn't good enough."

BUD: (As the father) I did the best I could even if it wasn't good enough.

BOYNE: Be the boy.

BUD: I'm glad. I'm glad to hear what you just said. At least I know there was some feeling there but you just couldn't show it.

BOYNE: Now your father has to leave in a very, very short time. I want you to make your final statement to him and then say good-bye.

BUD: Dad, I never hated you. (He begins to sob.)

BOYNE: What is the rest of it?

BUD: There was so many times I wanted to be like you.

BOYNE: Say, "Sometimes I hated the way you treated me."

BUD: Sometimes I hated the way you treated me.

BOYNE: "But I always looked up to you and wanted to be like you."

BUD: I always looked up to you and wanted to be like you. I wanted them to know that my dad had a good mind and he had a tremendous memory.

BOYNE: Say that to him.

BUD: Dad, I want you to know I thought you had a great mind and a tremendous memory—one thing that I always wanted.

BOYNE: All right. Make your final statement to him and say good-bye.

BUD: Dad, I know you're going and before you go, I want you to know I love you.

BOYNE: Say good-bye.

BUD: Good-bye, Dad.

BOYNE: Be the father. Speak to your son now as you get ready to go.

BUD: (As the father) Son, it's been a hell of a life. I've waited a long time to hear you say those words. I'm sorry they had to come now, but it's not too late. I'm glad to hear them.

BOYNE: Is there anything that you want to leave with your son, any suggestions, information about his life, things he should hope for in life or look for and expect to find? Give him some fatherly advice now before you say good-bye and go.

BUD: (As the father) Son, I don't want you to copy me. I've sinned many times, and if I've got some good qualities, that's the one thing I want to leave to you. But don't try to mimic me, don't try to copy my life. Don't try to pattern your life after me—just go ahead and do the best you can.

BOYNE: Do you think that he may find someone to love him?

BUD: (As the father) Son, I'm going, getting ready to go, and I want you to know that there's someone in this lifetime, in your lifetime that's going to love you very much. You're a decent man.

BOYNE: Say good-bye to your son.

BUD: (As the father) Good-bye, Son.

BOYNE: (Gil places his hand on Bud's forehead as he says) Let your mind grow clear. Come up to this time and place. (Gil has his hand on Bud's head, rocking it a bit.) Repeat after me. "I now forgive everyone who has ever harmed me in any way."

BUD: I now forgive everyone who has ever harmed me in any way.

BOYNE: "I wish for them the same good I wish for myself."

BUD: I wish for them the same good that I wish for myself.

BOYNE: "I bless them with my love."

BUD: I bless them with my love.

BOYNE: "I now forgive myself for every mistake that I've ever made."

BUD: I now forgive myself for every mistake that I've ever made.

BOYNE: "I see each mistake as a stepping stone."

BUD: I see each mistake as a stepping stone.

BOYNE: "To greater understanding and greater opportunity."

BUD: To greater understanding and to greater opportunities.

BOYNE: "I freely forgive as I would be forgiven."

BUD: I freely forgive as I would be forgiven.

BOYNE: Take your mind and go into, through your body. When you've done that, give a report on what you're experiencing.

BUD: Peace—I'm not tense. I feel refreshed. I feel relaxed.

BOYNE: (Gil takes a hold of Bud's right hand and places his left hand on Bud's forehead.) Let your mind grow clear. Now, Bud, there are things in life for you to do that can and should be done better by you than by any other person. You're important to life. Never before has there been any other person on this planet exactly like you, for if there had been, there wouldn't be any need for you to be here. Never again will there be another person on this planet exactly like you, for if there were going to be, there would be no need for you to be here. Bud, from this time forward, you begin to accept yourself as a lovable person because you are lovable. You now begin to accept yourself as a lovable person. You like people. You enjoy being with people. You enjoy the company of people. You enjoy being in a social gathering. Bud, people are aware that you like them. People like to talk to you, and people like to listen to you. People enjoy your company. Bud, you're a lovable person.

You look upon each new woman that you meet as a possible friend. When you meet a woman, you communicate to her that you like women. You enjoy being with a special woman. As you continue to increase your circle of friendships, you now know that sooner or later you'll meet a woman with whom you can form a loving relationship, a woman who will feel close to you and you to she. Bud, your mother is very advanced in years. You have many years to live, but the years of your mother may be very short and you've indicated that senility is coming upon her and her mental life is already approaching it's end. Bud, there are people in the world who have love to give and you're now going to become eager and willing to accept the love, affection, and approval that's available to you now. With each passing day, it becomes easier for you to express love and affection, and you do it by paying compliments, by making contact with people, by doing good and kind things for others, and you'll find this is quite easy for you to do. Each time you relax like this, these ideas will filter up from deeper levels of your subconscious mind.

With each passing day, you feel yourself being transformed. You know, Paul said, "Be ye transformed by the renewing of your mind," and that's what you're doing now. It doesn't take very long, for he said, "Be ye transformed in the twinkling of an eye." When you open your eyes, you're going to feel that you are a new man. You've put aside childish things. You're going to feel a great sense of lightness, as if a great weight has come off your shoulders now. Now, Bud, if you met a child that had been very severely mistreated and needed a friend, you'd now know how to take care of that child. In the same way, we're going to ask that critical parent inside you to become a nurturing parent. Bud, to have you begin to be good to yourself, to love yourself, to appreciate yourself. Are you now willing to do that, Bud?

BUD: Yes.

BOYNE: One of the ways that you can appreciate yourself is that you can now begin to cut down on the use of alcohol, because you know the kind of peace that you're experiencing now, the peace that surpasses understanding, is not to be found in a bottle, is it?

BUD: That's right.

BOYNE: Now in just a few moments I'm going to have you open your eyes. Before I do, is there anything further that you want to say to me or ask me or tell me for today?

BUD: I just want to say my dad wasn't always mean.

BOYNE: Of course he wasn't.

BUD: Just at times he made us mind.

BOYNE: Now that you understand, you can feel these loving feelings for your father flooding in and filling you, can't you?

BUD: Yes.

BOYNE: Isn't that a wonderful feeling to feel that love?

BUD: Yes, it is and I would like to say that I wish I had his mind and his memory.

BOYNE: I think that you have genetically inherited many of the good attributes and strengths of your father. But let's test it out, because I think your perception is not quite accurate. How are you like your father? In what ways are you like your father?

BUD: Well, he made a home.

BOYNE: He provided for his family and you provided for your family.

BUD: Yes.

BOYNE: That's good. There are a lot of men in this world that don't provide for their wife and family. How else are you like your father?

BUD: Well, he wasn't a man that got into trouble. He drank.

BOYNE: But he was law-abiding.

BUD: Yes.

BOYNE: And you're law-abiding.

BUD: Yes.

BOYNE: How else are you like your father?

BUD: If he knew or if he thought that there was one of us or all three of us that had to have something, he'd bust his back to get it for us. He was that kind of a man.

BOYNE: He took care of his children.

BUD: I would do the same thing.

BOYNE: And you've taken care of your children.

BUD: Yes.

BOYNE: Sounds like your father was a very responsible father and parent.

BUD: He was. He was strict and like I said, he had a short temper. I can remember two or three instances when he really laced it to me.

BOYNE: You've forgiven him for that now, haven't you?

BUD: Absolutely.

BOYNE: Sure. How are you unlike—different from your father?

BUD: Well, he had a better mind than I've got. I can't think of anybody that ever beat him in any kind of a deal. And it seems like I'm getting beat all the time.

BOYNE: Well that's the way you've behaved. That doesn't necessarily mean that's your mind. My appraisal and my observation of the way your mind has worked here with me is that you have a good, clear, sharp, functioning mind that works for you. I think you've deluded yourself over a long period of time, based on this comparison with your father that you're not so bright. You've learned to play dumb, and I'm going to ask you as you start being good to yourself, just give up that habit of playing dumb. Can you do that?

BUD: I'm going to work on it.

BOYNE: All right. How else are you different from your father?

BUD: Well, I don't know. I don't have the temper that he has. I'm easygoing.

BOYNE: That's a strength that you have—his temper got him into trouble a lot of times, didn't it?

BUD: Yes, yes.

BOYNE: Although sometimes when you were upset as a child, your temper came up and you just reached out and punched somebody, didn't you?

BUD: Yes, I did.

BOYNE: So you've learned to control your temper.

BUD: Yes, I have.

BOYNE: And your father never did learn to control his.

BUD: Not that I ever could remember.

BOYNE: So there are similarities and there are differences. Your father was his man, and you are your man.

BUD: Yes, yes.

BOYNE: For you are you and he was he.

BUD: That's right.

BOYNE: He did his thing, and you can do your thing.

BUD: That's right.

BOYNE: Before I bring you up, is there anything further you want to say to me or ask me or tell me?

BUD: No.

BOYNE: All right. Quickly now, who do I remind you of?

BUD: John Barrymore.

BOYNE: John Barrymore. That's very complimentary because John was a great actor and had a great romantic appeal. How am I like John Barrymore?

BUD: Your profile and his are almost identical.

BOYNE: What qualities do I share with John Barrymore or any of the roles that he played?

BUD: Well, he gave the appearance of being a forceful man and I think that you have the same qualities.

BOYNE: All right. I am going to count from one up to five. At the count of five, eyelids open, fully aware, feeling wonderful. One, slowly, calmly, easily, gently returning to your full awareness once again. Two, each muscle and nerve in your body is loose and limp and relaxed, and you feel good. Three, from head to toe, Bud, you feel wonderfully good in every way. On number four, your eyes begin to feel sparkling clear. On the next number now, eyelids open, fully aware, feeling wonderfully good. Number five, eyelids open now. Take a deep breath. Fill up your lungs and stretch. Well, you kind of went through the wringer that time, didn't you?

BUD: I really did. (He looks much happier and full of life and confidence.)

BOYNE: And came out on the other side.

BUD: (He laughs.)

BOYNE: You sure surprised yourself, didn't you?

BUD: I didn't think I could go through with it.

BOYNE: You're a lot tougher than you thought you were. Tell me about this experience. What did you get out of it?

BUD: Well, you know, I don't have a great way with words or anything, but I'm just glad that I came here.

BOYNE: I am too, Bud, but with me at least, will you practice with me? Don't tell me what you don't have, just use what you do have.

BUD: All right.

BOYNE: What did you get out of all of this?

BUD: Well, there's no question about it. I'm much more relaxed and I can look at people differently. I found that out this morning in the restaurant, and when I came here, I didn't realize it, but I had hate in me. I wanted to reach out, and if I saw a face I didn't like I wanted to strike out at them. Now I feel real good, especially now. (He looks like a new person, full of confidence.)

BOYNE: Put your hand in mine. Look at me. This is very important, what I'm going to tell you now. You see, up until this moment, you have not been recognizing people. When you looked at them, you didn't see a human being. You saw a motion picture screen, and you played your funny little movies up on that screen. You know what they are?

BUD: (He nods in agreement.)

BOYNE: They are all the terribly critical thoughts that you held about yourself. You projected them out there and said, "Look at the rotten, vicious thoughts they are thinking about me." No wonder you hated them, but you see how unkind that was to them because that's not them at all. That's just a projection you put on them. In a moment, I'm going to have you stand up and look at each person and tell me what you see. It's going to be quite easy for you to do, and you're going to be surprised at what you see. Now first, look out at some of these faces that you can see. Focus on, look around. Tell me what it is that you see.

BUD: Friendly faces.

BOYNE: "I see friendship." Look again and tell me what it is that you see. Just look around.

BUD: Well, I just see people that I like.

BOYNE: "I feel a feeling of liking for these people." Now look around again and tell me what you see.

BUD: I think I see people that are with me.

BOYNE: Do you want to use a word to characterize that "with me"?

BUD: I might say, I don't—

BOYNE: Go ahead, take a chance.

BUD: Believe in me.

BOYNE: Look around again, and what is it that you see?

BUD: I think they believe me.

BOYNE: Look again. What is it that you see? I think you're starting to see it.

BUD: I see friends.

BOYNE: Look again and see if you can see more than friendship.

BUD: Love?

BOYNE: Well, you put a question mark after it. Look again.

BUD: I see love!

BOYNE: Welcome to the world, Bud!

BUD: Thank you.

AUDIENCE: (They applaud Bud.)

BOYNE: We make ourselves blind and we are unable and unwilling to see the love and approval that surrounds us all the time. So we alienate ourselves and keep ourselves away from the world and project that somehow they find us unlovable. It's a painful and difficult task to reveal ourselves, to become open, and to say, "Here I am, strengths and weaknesses. I hope you'll find some part of me to love. If not, well, then I can accept that too, for that's the way it is. There are others in the world who have love for me, to nourish me, and will encourage and excite me to express love that is nourishing to them, for love makes the world go round." Until the next time, this is Gil Boyne.

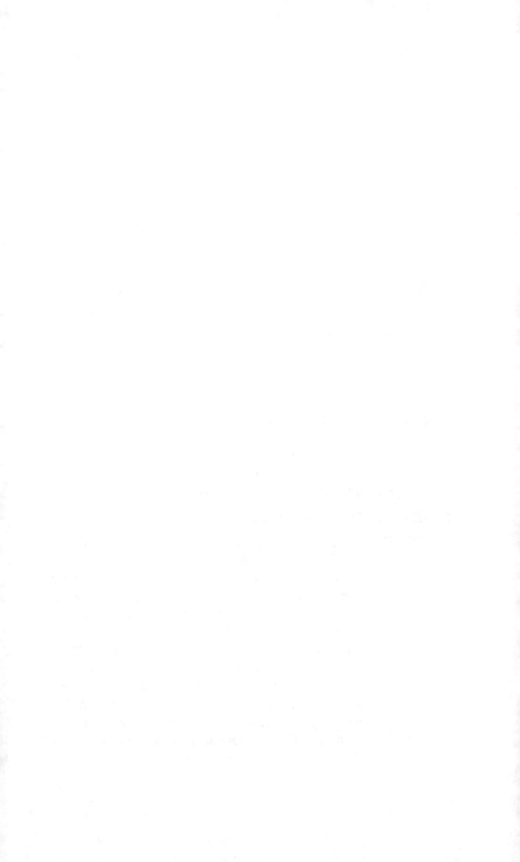

HYPNOTHERAPY TO CURE IMPOTENCE

The Case of Tyler ("I Can't Get It Up at the Right Time")

An attractive, twenty-year-old male reports an inability to achieve erection in sexually intimate situations.

Age regressions, abreaction, Gestalt dialogues, and extensive reeducation programming on two consecutive days create a psychic transformation.

One week later, Tyler reports that his problem is solved.

THE CASE OF TYLER
"I Can't Get It Up at the Right Time"
Session One

(BOYNE ADDRESSES THE AUDIENCE)

BOYNE: Hello. This is Gil Boyne, and welcome again to the Hypnotherapy Video Clinic. Today we're beginning a new case, and we're here with Tyler.

(BOYNE ADDRESSES TYLER)

How can I help you today?

TYLER: Well, actually I have two problems. My most serious one probably is girls. I like girls and everything, because I'm twenty and I'm in college and as I said, I like girls; but I kind of get scared with them when I'm out on a date and it's getting kind of intimate. I mean I've had sex with a girlfriend before, but I wasn't able to have sex with that girl until I really got comfortable with her. It was two or three different times, you know, that I failed. And, I've had a number of times where I met a girl, maybe the first time, a couple of weeks after just dating her and then, you know, not being able to get it up, and that really upsets me and I have no idea what to do about that at all.

BOYNE: All right. Let's start. How old were you when you had your first opportunity for some kind of sexual interaction with a female?

TYLER: Any kind of sexual interaction?

BOYNE: Other than just kissing on the lips.

TYLER: Oh, I was in seventh grade. About twelve or thirteen? My whole class was into playing with girls and going down into their pants and stuff like that.

BOYNE: That's a difficult time because you may remember when you were a certain age, five or six, and you and the other boys built a clubhouse and put a sign over it, "No girls allowed." Then slowly you moved beyond that stage and you began to discover the opposite sex does attract you and makes you interested, but you've got to bridge the fear gap. Some do it easier than others, and some for a great variety of reasons. Sometimes when there are sisters in the home, it makes it a bit easier because there's a little more understanding of what girls are like. How many children are in your family?

TYLER: There're four kids including me. All boys, including a twin.

BOYNE: So I lucked into it when I said it's easier when there are sisters in the home. Conversely, females are more exotic creatures when you know nothing about them.

TYLER: Yeah, I guess so.

BOYNE: (Laughter) So your problem is a common one. Now, where were you raised?

TYLER: In Kansas City.

BOYNE: So about the time you were twelve and the other fellows in the class were fiddling around and telling greatly exaggerated stories of what happened—

TYLER: (Laughter) Yeah! No kidding.

BOYNE: What happened to you?

TYLER: Oh, we were all playing around and I was playing around right along with them and there was a group of guys and a group of girls, you know. Those two groups would always get together on weekends and if not the whole group, parts of the group would. That happened for quite a long time, and I was always involved with that group.

BOYNE: What kind of "playing around"? Generally just touching, or did it also include intercourse?

TYLER: No, just touching, playing around.

BOYNE: What is sometimes referred to by young people as "making out."

TYLER: Yeah, and seeing how far you can get.

BOYNE: During that period of time, did you feel that your ability to make out was as good as any of the other fellows, or better than, or less than?

TYLER: I always felt about the same. I mean I had grown up all the way from kindergarten with most of the guys that were doing it anyway, and we had always been together for quite a long time.

BOYNE: You mentioned there were four of you in the family and you said you were a twin.

TYLER: Right.

BOYNE: Are your two other brothers older or younger?

TYLER: I have my twin brother and then there's one that is two years older than me and then there is one that is six years older than me.

BOYNE: Did either of those older brothers attempt to tell you the facts of life, either in a straight way or just kidding around?

TYLER: Well, the one that is two years older than me, Jeff, he's always been a ladies man. He's been into ladies for a long time. I was too young when he was at the point where girls weren't allowed, but he's always been a lady's man and he's always had dates. Also, talking to my mom, "You're going to drive me to get into dates," or whatever. Even up to when I was in seventh grade and he was in ninth grade. He was a big lady's man at the same junior high school that I was in, you know. He was kind of a big guy there, you know, because he was supposed to be tough and a big man in school. You understand what I am saying?

BOYNE: Yes.

TYLER: I mean, he was always having girls, talking about them, and many of his friends would come over and they would bug Tom and I about it, jump on us and say, "Have you ever?" you know, and start kind of hitting us and stuff like that.

BOYNE: You mean, ask you, "Are you still a cherry?" and that kind of thing.

TYLER: (Laughter) Yeah, basically.

BOYNE: Tell you about all their great exploits. How did you feel during that period of time?

TYLER: Well, I always looked up to Jeff. I thought he was a real neat guy and everything. I'd always looked forward to jumping further into the girl scene. And then, because he was always going out and, you know, getting drunk, and it was kind of a big thing to get drunk and be with the girls and stuff. I always thought it would be neat to do that when I get a little bit older.

BOYNE: Did either of your brothers ridicule you or make you feel like the kid brother is kind of clumsy around girls?

TYLER: Well, they did a little bit when we were all alone but nothing really bad. If we were out in public they were always sticking up for us no matter what.

BOYNE: Do you recall anything your mother might have had to say about your brothers' skirt-chasing activities?

TYLER: She was always agreeing with everything. All four of us just live with my mom. My dad hadn't lived with us for a long time, and she would always agree with us. She didn't care if, when we were real little we looked at naked ladies and pictures and everything because she said, "That's great, that's natural." Whatever actions we took, she accepted it.

BOYNE: She didn't say that's disrespectful to women or anything like that?

TYLER: Well, if we got a little dirty and, you know, joking around and stuff, she'd kind of crack down on that.

BOYNE: You said your father wasn't around for a long time. Where was he?

TYLER: He lived about fifteen or twenty minutes away, which was a long way considering none of us could drive except for my oldest brother, and he wasn't around that much to drive. And that was from the beginning of my twelfth year until like last year.

BOYNE: Did he and your mother agree to live apart?

TYLER: Yes, they separated.

BOYNE: Did he continue to support the family?

TYLER: Yes, very much so.

BOYNE: And did he come to visit you and your brothers?

TYLER: Well, we more or less went down there to visit with him, and he would take us out and occasionally he would come to the house and stuff.

BOYNE: Did he have female friends?

TYLER: Yes, he had one main girlfriend.

BOYNE: Did she live there with him?

TYLER: No.

BOYNE: When you went to see him, was she there with him?

TYLER: Not for a long time. He didn't let us see her, not for a long time. But we knew he had a girlfriend.

BOYNE: Did your mother ever talk about his woman friend?

TYLER: She'd always get real pissed at him because, they had had an affair, and that's one of the main reasons he moved out. They were supposed to have gotten back together. Now they were just living apart because they were thinking about trying to get back together, but I don't think the trying was really good.

BOYNE: Reconciliation never came about, but your mother remained angry because she felt rejected for this other woman.

TYLER: I think so at first, and then it came to the point where she didn't even want us kids seeing her at all around my father, at least for a long time.

BOYNE: Do you remember if you or your brothers or your twin had any discussions about this other woman or your dad's behavior toward her? That maybe it was just a sexual attraction that pulled him to her, that pulled him away from your mother, or it would have been better if he had stayed? Do you ever remember discussing it?

TYLER: I think I remember him saying that he liked this other woman because she was more of a housewife to him and my mother was always real independent. She didn't want to stay home and cook and stuff. She wanted to go out and paint and go out and kind of hit the town and stuff. She was more an independent woman. He always thought that, you know, if he brought home the paycheck, then he would have somebody to take care of him. So basically I remember talk like that.

BOYNE: Did you feel you loved your father?

TYLER: Oh, yes.

BOYNE: And he loved you?

TYLER: Oh, yes. I think all of us kids were the main thing in his life for a long time. He wouldn't even marry this other lady until we're all out of the house.

BOYNE: So you characterize him as a good father.

TYLER: Very much so.

BOYNE: A good and loving father. All right. Let's go to the first time that you had this difficulty, when fear, anxiety, and tension inhibited your sexual function, inhibited your erection. Can you recall that time?

TYLER: I think so. The first time was when I was in ninth grade and there was this girl in seventh grade. We were dating, and it was kind of like we were the big couple in school, you know, because she was real cute and I guess I was kind of like pretty high up on the totem pole in school.

BOYNE: Were you an athlete?

TYLER: Yes, I was, and, you know, everyone said, "Asha and Tyler look good together." We had always gone far but we hadn't gone all the way. Then finally one time we were at my house and we were going to try, and we got each other's clothes off, and it took off from there. But I don't know, too much excitement or something and I couldn't get it up and it really upset me.

BOYNE: Now you said, "Too much excitement really upset me." Does "too much excitment" mean "I ejaculated before I penetrated," or "I had an erection and lost it," or "I didn't develop an erection when I wanted to"?

TYLER: Number Three—I didn't develop an erection when I wanted to. But see, what's weird is, you know, all the times before when we had played around, I had an erection.

BOYNE: At that time did your mother or did anyone ever talk to you about being careful, you know, not to get married too soon. "Be careful, a lot of fellows get girls pregnant and they're married before they know it, and then they are working in some kind of a job with no future" and so on?

TYLER: No, I think that she thought that Tom, my twin brother, and I were too young at the time to even be that close to girls. I think she was always yelling at Chas, my oldest brother, because he had a girlfriend, and he wasn't too responsible.

BOYNE: What does that mean?

TYLER: He was always wrecking the family car, and he was always getting in trouble. He wasn't too responsible. And Jeff was just wild but my parents knew that he was kind of smart and knew better than to do something foolish, but he was always really wild.

BOYNE: Your older brother, the one six years older, is he married?

TYLER: Yes, the one six years older than me is married now.

BOYNE: Do you know if there was a pregancy at the time of marriage?

TYLER: No, she kind of made him marry her because they dated for five years before then.

BOYNE: I see. So you suspect that one day she said to him, "Either you name the day or look elsewhere."

TYLER: That's right. I know that. At least that's the way she brags at me all the time.

BOYNE: Well, she did the right thing. That's what women traditionally do after such a long relationship—to bring it to a head.

TYLER: Whenever I have a girlfriend, she always sits down right next to me and starts going, "Well, when's the day?" or "Come on, are you guys getting real serious or what?" Because she's the only girl in our family and she has five brothers herself. So, she's the only girl in this huge family of boys.

BOYNE: At family get-togethers, holiday dinners and so on, there she sits, like a queen.

TYLER: Yeah. She's always going on, "Come on, when am I going to get a sister-in-law?"

BOYNE: Does your mother speak well of and seem to like your sister-in-law?

TYLER: They live in the same apartment complex right next to each other so they're always down there talking and everything.

BOYNE: When this experience happened and you experienced an inhibition on your erection, how did that affect you? First, what happened to your lady friend? What was her attitude toward it?

TYLER: Oh, I don't know. I don't really remember.

REPRESSION

BOYNE: Do you remember if she was at all critical: "Hey, what's wrong?" or "Don't you like me?" or made some other kind of a statement: "That's all right, there will always be another time," or "Just forget about it"?

TYLER: I don't really remember what she said, but I think she was more hostile toward me than anything else.

BOYNE: Well, that's appropriate because you've been aroused before with her, and now it comes down to "this is the time." She's made a decision, and you're going to carry this level of intimacy into a fuller level of physical intimacy, and she can interpret that nonerection as meaning that you really don't care for her that much. That is, she doesn't excite you that much and that can be upsetting to her, and one way of dealing with it is to be hostile like, "What the heck's the matter with you anyway? What kind of a guy are you?"

TYLER: I have had another girlfriend that's done that too.

BOYNE: It's based on their own insecurity. So the first thing I'm going to tell you now, today, is this: From now on whenever you are alone with a female and it might develop into something of an intimate, physical nature and before you head for the bedroom, this is what you are to do. You say, "Before we go into that bedroom, I want to tell you something. I have had a bit of a problem. I'm working on it, and I feel sure that I'll soon be over it. I'm only telling you about it because if for any reason I don't show powerful desire for you physically, it doesn't mean that I am not excited by you. It doesn't mean that I don't care about you, and it doesn't mean that I don't find you attractive and exciting. It is my problem and I'm working on it." The moment you do that, all the fear and anxiety that you have about, "Am I going to make it?" will disappear because now you've been up front with her.

Now, on the other hand, let me tell you the kinds of responses you might get. It's conceivable that a female might say, "Well, let's not go into the bedroom. Let's wait awhile until you solve the problem."

AUDIENCE: (Laughter)

TYLER: That's what I would be afraid of.

BOYNE: Sure, but that's the most unlikely response. Generally they feel kind of relieved. They feel empathetic. One man told me when he said that, the woman replied "Just leave everything to me. I'll take care of everything." He said that sure enough, she did.

AUDIENCE: (Laughter)

TYLER: Around my age, when you go to bars like that, not many girls are going to want to hear that. They'll always come back hostile and stuff. Especially the one-night stands.

BOYNE: The woman I just described, she was an older woman. She was about thirty-five and had a greater understanding of men.

TYLER: Well, I had dated this girl for a couple of weeks because I liked her and she was real cute and everything, but I had talked to her about it first. There wasn't any problem, you know, because I kind of forgot about it before it had happened. But some of the girls that I pick up on, I don't want them to have the satisfaction of knowing that I couldn't get it up or something. So, usually, I'll just sit there and say, "Well, I guess I was too drunk." I know it's a cop out for me but...

BOYNE: There's another thing I want to say to you, my friend. As a young man comes into your age, there is often a feeling expressed by his peers that "ass is ass if it's on a cow," and if it's available, you've got to get some. This attitude completely ignores the fact that men are just as sensitive and selective as females are. And even though there's this time of great sexual desire and the mind is filled with sexual ideas day and night, it's just not really that way. Despite the sexual frenzy that comes with the outpouring of those hormones, many males really have a kind of a sensitivity and a selectivity that they're not even aware of. When they meet the gal in the bar and she shows some interest, it's out to the back of the van. But, there's a part of him that really doesn't want to get that intimate so quickly with this particular person, or maybe there's something about her that is really turning him off at the psychic level. It might be the way she talks, the way she looks, the kind of thoughts she's expressing. But she has a cute bottom or a great set of bazooms.

TYLER: That's what I don't understand. I don't see why something like that wouldn't turn me on no matter how she was.

BOYNE: You see, that's what I'm talking about. That's the propaganda that you and most of us came to swallow—that if we're "macho men," then we'll screw a snake if someone will hold its head.

TYLER: (Laughter)

BOYNE: That's not the way it is forevermore. It wasn't for me, and I've learned from working with many men that it's not really that way. So, that's one thing I want you to consider, that you're not just a rutting bull in heat that sniffs the secretion of some other animal and is going to mate with it no matter what. You're much more than that.

TYLER: Oh, I think that I am. Like I prefer to have a girlfriend more than being able to go out and get laid. But girlfriends don't come easy, you know.

BOYNE: Right. What you're saying is you want a relationship with a girl who's more than just a sexual outlet. That's different from the one-nighter. You pick her up in the bar and bang, that's it and after it's all over, you say, "Well, that's the end of that." There's sex with relationship. You get to know each other, and you go out one night a week and sooner or later you get to it, and regularly you get to it again. Then there's sex with relationship that leads to commitment. You go steady, then you become engaged and maybe even live together and/or get married. Now you can participate in and enjoy sex at all of those levels, depending on the circumstances. But you do have preferences, and as a young single male, your preference is relationship because you know the old saying "I want someone I can talk to and listen to after I get out of bed."

AUDIENCE: (Laughter)

BOYNE: And when you're with someone you really don't like and you're hearing that inane prattle, you think "Oh, do I have to listen to this? Is this the price I have to pay just because we had a little sex in bed together? Now I have to put up with this?" You know there are levels of preference other than "I prefer a girl with a big chest, a nicely rounded bottom, or pretty legs."

TYLER: Yeah, but I would like to enjoy that until I found a girlfriend.

BOYNE: You see, that's the paradox that you're trying to resolve. So all that you remember about this experience is that this young woman became hostile. She said, "Hey, Charlie, what is this?"

TYLER: Well, she didn't ever get really hostile. It's just the words that she would say, you know. She'd say, "What's your problem?" She just said a few things in a nice, easy voice. I was only fifteen I guess. She was two years younger than me, and after that she acted like "It's no big deal with me," and so and so did it with her, which I knew was a lie then because she was just making it up to get back at me. You know, she just kind of admitted that she had done it with a couple of other guys.

BOYNE: How did you feel when you heard all that information?

TYLER: Like "that's a crock of shit, and why the hell would I care."

BOYNE: (Laughter) You were right in feeling that as hostility. That said to you, "You're not so special, Charlie. I make it with others too, you know, and they find me exciting!"

TYLER: I think that was the beginning of the end, and then, what really made me mad was a few weeks later, there's a guy that I had grown up with. I found out that they slept together the night after we broke up. The girl and I broke up and then she went and had sex with this other guy, and I know it was just to spite me because we broke up I knew she was going to do something like that. I had a female friend and we played around but we didn't do anything close like that. Of course, I lied and told her that we went pretty far and stuff.

BOYNE: (Laughter) More game playing.

TYLER: Of course, I mean, I was only fifteen, I had to play games, or I'd feel real bad.

BOYNE: You know quite often the young women that seem to

be quite caught up in being sexually active are really acting out a deeper feeling within. It's a feeling of being unlovable. They are trying to resolve their adolescent rebellion at home. And my experience in working as a counselor is that many of them reported that during those adolescent years, they were very sexually active and had little or no sexual gratification; which means they had little or no sensation in their genitals. What they really wanted was the closeness. They said what they enjoyed most was the kissing, sometimes a bit of breast and nipple stimulation, but as the action moved downward, there was less and less response. What they wanted most in that moment was to feel needed, to see him excited, hear him say, "I love you," or "You're the greatest," or "I've got to have you," or whatever it was. What is inappropriately termed "promiscuity" or "sexual activity" in females is quite often just the reverse. It's not a sign that that person is highly sexual. It's often a sign that they just have deep-rooted feelings of being unlovable, and they're trying to overcome that feeling in this way. Did you ever have that thought?

TYLER: Not really.

BOYNE: Will you think about it from time to time because it really is an exploitation, you know. When I was a young fellow, someone would say, "I'm going to tell you about a hot number. She puts out real easy." I look back now and feel sad because she wasn't hot and she wasn't putting out. She was just reaching out to try to find some reassurance that she was lovable to someone for a moment. I wish I could have had an uncle or someone who could have maybe tried to tell me that, so that I could have been a little bit helpful in a meaningful way.

TYLER: That is what I kept saying, when I told my father the problem and he said, "All men go through that same thing." For a while I thought it was that, you know, it kept happening.

BOYNE: There is a principle at work. When dealing with your subconscious mind, the greater the conscious effort, the less the subconscious response. That means if you have difficulty going to sleep, the harder you try to go to sleep, the more wide awake you become. You know that's true. Why? Well, because you can't go to sleep. You have to let sleep come upon you. In the same way you can't order yourself to have an erection. Believe it or not!

TYLER: I believe it, man.

BOYNE: When you experience an erection, it's a response to a stimulus either external or internal or both. What happens is that sometimes, because of too much to drink, anxiety, tension, fear, you can't function.

Let me tell a story. A scene just flashed in my mind. I was about twelve years old and this little girl lived with her mother and her sister in an apartment house upstairs from our apartment. Linda was very cute, and one day her mother went out to work and my mother and father went out to the movies and they hired her as a babysitter. I remember my sister was ten years younger—I guess my sister was two. There we were, and Linda said, "Let's play Mommy and Daddy. I'll be the mommy, you be the daddy, and she'll be our baby." Now there was a double bed and she put my little sister on a little army cot along side the bed, and she lay down and she said, "I'm the mommy, you're the daddy, you lay on top of me." I remember I lay on top of her, and I started shaking and my whole body was just trembling all over. She coached me and guided me through it, but it wasn't a very successful experience. I remember that shaking and trembling, and I kept saying to myself "I got to stop shaking," and the more I said, "I've got to stop," the more my body shook.

BUILDING RAPPORT BY REVELATION OF SIMILAR EXPERIENCE

Well, let's go back to this issue. For whatever reason, once you fail to get an erection you say, "Gee, will that happen the next time too?"

TYLER: (He nods in agreement.)

BOYNE: Now you begin to program it through fear. "That which I have feared has come upon me." When we picture in our mind that which we don't want to happen, it is a way of programming it to happen. In short, it becomes a self-fulfilling prophecy. The question, "Will that happen to me?" becomes a statement, "I'm afraid it will happen to me again," and the emotion connected with the fear is the major factor that causes it to happen again.

TYLER: (He nods in agreement.)

BOYNE: Here's the principle. Each time your nervous system reacts in a given way, it becomes easier for it to react that way the next time. That's what a habit is all about because it becomes easier for your nervous system to process that energy the same way every time. The proof of it is that if you really had anything organically wrong with you, then you wouldn't get erections at all.

TYLER: (He nods in agreement.)

BOYNE: You wouldn't get erections when you wake up in the morning, and you wouldn't get them after you're comfortable with a gal and know her for a few weeks.

TYLER: (He nods in agreement.)

BOYNE: Sometimes that problem is connected with the fear of rejection or feelings of sexual inadequacy.

TYLER: Or to impress this girl.

BOYNE: Wanting her to think, "Boy, he's a real stud. He's a great lover," or the need to compare yourself against others. Often when a young man becomes aware that this gal has been sexually active, he's afraid that she's going to rate him. If she's been with seven other guys, he fears that he's going to rate down at the bottom, the eighth; but actually it's not like an athletic competition. It's not how far can you throw the shot-put and measure the distance, because each time it's a relationship. Each time the experience has a unique quality. It should have a quality that's unique to the people involved. There's a magical chemistry that creates something between them. Unless it's purely hormonal, unless it's the irritation of the genitals and nothing more. You see, this thing got hard on me, and I have to do something with it, and she's here and that's better than a pound of liver in a mayonnaise jar.

TYLER: (Laughter)

BOYNE: Did you ever read *Portnoy's Complaint?*

TYLER: No.

BOYNE: No. When you leave here, I want you to go to the library and get this book, *Portnoy's Complaint.* It will help you to understand your sexuality better than you have before. It's about a young man and his problems with his sexuality and that's one of the things he talks about during his intense masturbation phase. So now this habit is with you and it's become worse?

TYLER: Uh-huh. Very much so. It makes me not even want to talk to girls when I go to bars with friends.

BOYNE: You find ways to back off. You find ways to withdraw?

TYLER: Uh-huh.

BOYNE: You say, "Well, she's not so hot," or "I've seen better." That kind of thing.

TYLER: (He nods in agreement)

BOYNE: All right. What brought you to me?

TYLER: My mom has always been into self-help and stuff like that, and my dad has a real good friend who's a psychiatrist, and I went to him a couple of times. I had asked him about hypnosis, and he said, "Oh, that doesn't work, but I can help you."

BOYNE: (Laughter) Did he help you?

TYLER: No, not at all. So I left and then one day I was home, and I was bumming out. So I said, "Hey, what the heck." I looked up in the yellow pages and I went to a hypnotist. The hypnotist saw me five times and the first time I don't remember being hypnotized, but it was an hour and a half later when I woke up. The next time I could understand what was going on. I don't know if I was hypnotized, and I think the other time I was hypnotized again. He made tapes for me and it didn't help at all.

BOYNE: How did you feel about him as a person?

TYLER: I liked him a lot. He was a real nice guy.

BOYNE: How old?

TYLER: I'd say he was early thirties. Real nice guy.

BOYNE: How did you feel about his capacity to relate to women at a sexual level? You called your brother a ladies man. Do you think that fellow was ever a ladies man?

TYLER: No.

BOYNE: No.

TYLER: (Laughter. Gil and Tyler shake hands.)

BOYNE: All right. Do you think that's connected to your lack of result with him?

TYLER: It could be. I've talked to my mom and she said, "Well, talk to Jeff," you know, he's a ladies man and everything. I look up to him. There's no way I'd talk to him about it. He'd go, "What? You can't what? What's the deal?" He would eventually help me but I'd get a lot of guff about it. Well, as I was saying, I was lead to you by my mom—she gave me a book on self-hypnosis. So I started reading it and your name came up quite a few times in it. So then I just called to get some information, and I was sent a big packet of information and also this school catalog about institute training. I'd always wanted to come to the institute training and everything but it cost a lot, I had to save up some money. In the meantime I would call up for tapes, and I got three of your tapes on Self-Confidence, Memory, and Relaxation. I listened to self-confidence for quite awhile, about a week or so, but I'm not too patient. I had thought hypnosis was that you don't remember anything, but last night and today the students here told me that you can be aware of everything that is going on.

BOYNE: Did this hypnotist give you any kind of tests to indicate that you were indeed hypnotized?

TYLER: Not that I know of. He told me one time that he had me make my finger real stiff, and he said that I did, but I don't recall him doing it. He was one of those dudes that graduated from college with this Ph.D. He had to use a flashing light and everything.

BOYNE: What you're experiencing is called "secondary impotence," secondary meaning it's not primary. Primary means you don't ever get an erection; secondary means you do, but not always at the right time. It is one of the simpliest problems for a skilled hypnotherapist who understands male sexuality. Secondary impotence doesn't usually show up in young males because there's such a powerful hormonal drive, or maybe young males just don't go to a therapist. Maybe they're too embarrassed until they're older. Generally males will come in from age thirty-five and older. In fact, tomorrow morning I'm going to show the class a film of a fifty-four-year-old man who suffers secondary impotence, and he's cured in three sessions. If you'll be here tomorrow, you'll see that tape. The reason it can be cured so easily is that it's natural for you to respond to appropriate stimulus. A young, strong, virile, powerful, healthy male responds in a certain way to sexual excitement.

One more question before I hypnotize you. Let me create a situation and you tell me which of these scenarios fits you. You're in a living room and you have a good strong erection. Now you head for the bedroom or lie down on the couch or start undressing and you lose it. That's one. You're in a living room and you're engaging in various kinds of genital, sexual stimulation and you're very aroused. You try to penetrate the female's vagina and you lose your erection. Number three: you don't get aroused when you are alone, even in the living room. And number four: you get aroused, ejaculate before you ever penetrate or just as you begin to, and it's all over for you. Which of those scenarios fits you, your circumstance?

TYLER: A combination of the first three. The fourth one didn't have anything to do with it.

BOYNE: Never experienced that premature ejaculation?

TYLER: (He shakes his head negatively.)

BOYNE: All right.

TYLER: One of the first times I really did it, I came awfully quick.

BOYNE: You had probably been fiddling around for hours. The prostate gland is shaped like a chestnut, and it fills up with fluid and the semen comes up from the testicles, then is stored in the prostate and mixes with this fluid. The nerve endings are in the head of your penis and they don't have to be stimulated by physical pressure. The stimulation can come from your psychic response, which means the way you feel about what's going on. But, when you reach a certain level of nervous excitement, these smooth involuntary muscles squeeze down on the prostate, and that's just like squeezing the rubber ball on the end of a syringe. When it squeezes, that triggers your ejaculation, you see.

TYLER: (He nods in agreement.)

BOYNE: All right. Are you ready for me to hypnotize you, my friend? Stand up. Take a step forward now and pull your feet together and just stand relaxed. SLEEP! Turn loose now. Relax. Let a good, pleasant feeling come all across your body. Let each muscle and nerve grow loose and limp and relaxed. The more I rock you, the deeper into hypnosis you're going. Now listen carefully, I'm going to tilt your head back and as I do, I'm going to count from five down to one and your eyelids lock so tightly closed (Gil's finger presses between Tyler's eyes) that the more you try to open them, the tighter they are locking closed.

Five, eyelids pressing down tightly. Four, they're pressing down and sealing shut. Three, sealing as if they were glued. Two, they're locked. The more you try to open them now, the tighter they're locking closed. One, try to open your eyelids. You see, they're stuck tight. Now you can stop trying. Relax and just sleep deeply. Make no further effort. That's good. Now you're breathing deeply and relaxing more with each easy breath that you take. I am going to walk you forward now and as I give you instructions, you can move easily. Take a step forward. That's it. Another step. Now I'm going to turn your body and move you back until you feel the edge of the couch against the back of your legs. As I push you down into this chair, you go down much deeper into hypnosis. Now go right on down and go much deeper. Lean back, balance yourself comfortably and go even deeper. That's fine. I'm going to take your hand and pull you forward a little bit. That's it.

Now sit once again. That's good. Now you can lean back, and you are comfortable now as you lean back. That's good.

Here's what we're going to do. I'm going to count from one up to twenty and as I do a light, easy, pleasant feeling moves into your right hand and into your right arm. As I continue counting that feeling grows stronger and stronger, and soon you'll feel the first slight movement, slight movement of the fingers, twitching of the muscles. Then your hand begins to lift and your arm begins to lift, and it continues moving, lifting and rising until it comes to rest over on your body. When you feel that movement in your hand and in your arm, don't try to resist. You could resist if you chose to. That's not why you're here. Let your subconscious mind do its perfect work.

Number one, the first light, easy sensation moves into the finger tips of your right hand. Number two, the feeling is spreading around beneath the fingernails. On number three, it's moving up to the first joint of the fingers. Number four, spreading to the large knuckles across the back of the hand. Number five, moving all across the back of the hand now. On number six, spreading down into the thumb. On number seven, all through the palm of your hand. On number eight, I want you to think of your left hand now, by comparison, your left hand is beginning to feel very, very heavy. While on number nine, your right hand grows lighter and lighter with each number I count.

Number ten, that light sensation is into the wrist and from the finger tips all the way up to the wrist, your hand is light, light and free and lifting just as light as a feather floating in the breeze and even lighter, as light as a gas filled balloon. Just as a gas filled balloon will rise and float toward the ceiling, in the same way your right hand begins moving, lifting, rising, and floating, coming up, moving, lifting, rising, and floating. Number eleven, think of your left hand now. That left hand feels as though it were heavy and made of lead. While on number twelve, the light sensation is moving up your right arm. Thirteen, as it is spreading up toward your elbow, your hand begins moving, lifting, rising, and floating. Fourteen, moving into the elbow now. And on fifteen, from the finger tips all the way up to the elbow, your right hand is light and free and beginning to lift and moving up toward your chest. Just as light as a feather floating in the breeze, even lighter, as light as a gas filled balloon. Just as that gas filled balloon will rise and float toward the ceiling in the same way your right hand is coming up and moving up. On sixteen, your left hand now feels as though it were made of marble or stone or lead.

Seventeen, on the next three numbers now, I want you to see and imagine I'm screwing a pulley into the ceiling above your head. This is a red plastic pulley and there is a blue plastic rope that runs up through it and then down again. On the next three numbers I'm going to count, I'm going to tie a rope around your wrist. I'll pull down on my end, that will draw your hand right on up. Here we go. Number seventeen, I'm tying a rope around your wrist. Eighteen, I reach up and grasp my end, and nineteen, as I am pulling down, it's drawing your hand right on up. That's it. Now it's coming up and I'll reach up again and grasp my end of the rope, and I'll draw it right on down and as I do it's pulling your hand right up. That's it. (Tyler's right hand begins to move upward.) I reach up with my right hand, I grasp the rope again, and I pull it down slowly and it keeps drawing your hand right on up. Now since this pulley is over your head as I pull down and that rope is pulling it, it is also swinging it in. So it is soon going to come right on over and touch your chest. As I pull down, here it comes, higher, moving and lifting, coming up. And I'm pulling it even higher and swinging it toward your chest right on the pulley now. And I reach up once again and I'm pulling it down and I'm pulling it down and as I do, it is swinging in toward your chest. When it touches your chest, your left arm immediately feels so heavy, as though it were made of marble or stone, far too heavy to lift. So heavy that in fact even the thought of lifting it is more than you want to concern yourself with. Now your hand is coming down to rest upon your chest, and as it does, your left arm feels as though it were made of marble, stone, or lead. That right arm just drops limply down and as it does, that left arm feels as though even the very thought of lifting it is more than you want to concern yourself with. (Tyler is resting is right arm on his chest.) You may if you wish make an effort and try to lift the left arm, but it just seems like it is more than you even want to concern your mind or your muscles with. Make a try if you wish and discover that it just feels as though it were made of marble or stone or lead.

Now I want you to just relax. Make no further effort. Let your arm drop down limply. (Tyler's arm drops limply down to his lap.) Go much deeper. You see, when I use the word sleep, I do not mean the kind of sleep that you sleep at night. I am referring to a very pleasant state of mental and physical relaxation that you are experiencing at this very moment. The word *hypnosis* is formed from the word *Hypnos*—the Greek god of Sleep.

The original title was neurohypnosis, meaning the sleep of the nerves. I know that you are aware and hear me and understand me just as you know it. For if you couldn't hear me and couldn't understand me, then you couldn't respond to the good, creative ideas that I express to you. Now, I want you to be aware that there's no real rational reason for one arm to feel lighter than the other or the left hand to feel heavier than the other or for your eyelids not to open the very moment you make an effort to open them. (Gil lightly touches Tyler's forehead above his eyes.) The only reason that they are not responding or they are re-sponding in this way is that the part of your mind that evaluates ideas rationally, the part of your mind that says, "Well, both of my hands should feel exactly the same," or "I can open my eyes any time I think about it," that part of your mind is temporarily relaxed. You might consider it to be very much like a stereo system. You know there is a balance knob, a rheostat. When you turn the knob to the left then all of the sound appears to come out of the left speaker and the right speaker and the right circuit is quiet. Now that circuit hasn't disappeared. It's just temporarily inactive. If you change it and turn that rheostat around to the right, the right speaker is activated, and the left circuit and the left speaker are quiet. In the same way that part of your mind just steps aside, sits down in an easy chair, looks at what's going on and says, "My, my, isn't that interesting." Now you can understand the dual nature of your mind—how one part of your mind can just relax and watch the other part of your mind accepting and acting upon good, creative, powerful, and beneficial suggestions. You're going to have a full and complete understanding of hypnosis this time, perhaps for the first time in your experience.

Now I'm going to work with you tomorrow and we're going to take the final step in solving this problem for you fully and completely. Before I close down, is there anything further that you want to say to me, ask me or tell me? Very quickly now, who do I remind you of?

TYLER: Jeff.

BOYNE: How am I like Jeff, your brother? Jeff's the one you call "the ladies man," is that right?

TYLER: Cool.

BOYNE: How am I like Jeff? What qualities do we both share?

TYLER: You get what you want.

BOYNE: We set out sights for something, we go after it, and we get it—and so will you.

Ms When I count from one up to five, let your eyelids open, you're calm, rested, refreshed, relaxed, and you feel wonderfully good. One, slowly, calmly, easily, and gently returning to your full awareness once again. Two, each muscle and nerve in your body is loose and limp and relaxed. You feel wonderfully good, lighter than you have felt in years, on number three. Number four, on the next number your eyelids begin to feel sparkling clear, you're wonderfully relaxed, physically relaxed, mentally relaxed, emotionally calm and serene. On the next number, eyelids open, fully aware, feeling wonderfully good. Number five, eyelids open. Take a good deep breath. Fill up your lungs and stretch.

Well, you surprised yourself today, didn't you. (Gil and Tyler laugh as they shake hands.) Tell me about it.

TYLER: What's to tell?

BOYNE: Were you surprised to feel your hand lifting up like that?

TYLER: Yeah. At first I thought, when you were counting, you were getting into the teens and it wasn't moving. I thought, "Well, why isn't it moving?" and then you touched it like that, and I felt—where your fingers had touched I felt—that kind of pulling, so it was just going up.

BOYNE: Right, and when I stood you up and your eyelids stuck...

TYLER: They did feel stuck. At first, I was just like, "Well, if you know what's going on around you, you're not hypnotized." But then I remember the whole class saying that that doesn't matter.

BOYNE: You remember how heavy your arm felt?

TYLER: I sure did.

BOYNE: Now the other hypnotist didn't do any of those tests, did he?

TYLER: He didn't do anything.

BOYNE: I've got about thirty seconds and I want to finish this lesson to the class.

(BOYNE ADDRESSES THE AUDIENCE)

Last week I taught the members of this class that you must use these tests if you want to bring to the conscious mind an awareness of a trance state. And even after that was taught, someone else in the class came to me and said, "You know, I heard people out there that are reviewing this class, people that are in practice, say, 'Oh, that's all unnecessary. You don't have to do those tests.'" You'd better rethink it and you'd better rethink your own fear. You better find out why you're unwilling to persuade that person, to educate that person, to let them know what hypnosis really is because if you don't, they're not coming back.

(BOYNE ADDRESSES TYLER)

BOYNE: Have you been hypnotized today?

TYLER: Yeah. I think so. Yeah.

BOYNE: What made you think so?

TYLER: Well, I couldn't open my eyes.

BOYNE: We're going to finish this job tomorrow, and we're going to finish this case history and send this young man on his way so that he can live a full, free, happy expression of life that God and nature intended for him.

Until then, this is Gil Boyne.

THE CASE OF TYLER
"I Can't Get It Up at the Right Time"
Session Two

(BOYNE ADDRESSES AUDIENCE)

BOYNE: Hello, this is Gil Boyne. Welcome again to the Hypnotherapy Video Clinic. Today we're back with Tyler. We worked with him yesterday so let's pick up where we left off.

(BOYNE ADDRESSES TYLER)

Welcome. Tell me about your thoughts and feelings since your experience here yesterday.

TYLER: Well, I guess I'm a little scared, you know. I mean, I know your reputation, and I saw some of your work. I'm still kind of scared that it's not going to help me as much, but I still have faith.

BOYNE: So you have kind of mixed feelings. On one hand you say, "Well, I guess if I'm going to get a result, this is the place I'm going to get it." On the other hand, "Boy, I sure hope I don't miss it."

TYLER: That's about right.

BOYNE: You just finished seeing a film about a man who has similar problems and I worked with him very successfully, except it might have been more difficult for him because he was fifty-four.

TYLER: (He nods in agreement.)

BOYNE: What were your thoughts as you watched that film?

TYLER: Well, I was thinking I was basically the same. It was coming along the same. Then I was looking towards the end to see how it was going, and he was saying it was successful and everything, so I was real excited about that.

BOYNE: He said that if his condition was a one when he arrived, on a scale of one to ten, he was now eight and a half.

TYLER: (He nods in agreement.)

BOYNE: That's pretty good, isn't it? Was the method in which his problem was solved in any way as you thought hypnotherapy might be, or was it different, and if so, tell me the difference.

TYLER: Well, I've always had a basic idea of what hypnosis was, but ever since I've come down here, I've got to the point of what it really is. When I saw on the video was basically how you were teaching him how it really was, and it was working. So basically, it was coming to the point where I was believing, I guess.

BOYNE: What were your thoughts as you went to sleep last night in bed and were thinking this whole thing over?

TYLER: Well, I really didn't think anything at first, but I woke up in the middle of the night and started having really mixed suggestions. I mean my conscience was going over everything that was going on, and then when I went back to sleep, it was like I kept having dreams of being hypnotized. I kept having dreams of putting myself to sleep and going deeper and deeper into sleep. You know, I'd wake up and I'd roll over and say, "I'm too tired to get out of bed," and really enjoyed going back to sleep.

BOYNE: (Laughter) Is waking up in the middle of the night a customary thing for you?

TYLER: Very much so. Very much.

BOYNE: Do you ever walk in your sleep?

TYLER: No, I don't.

BOYNE: All right. Anything else that you want to talk about before I hypnotize you?

TYLER: I've become kind of scared of females. I think I probably told you already, but I wanted to make sure I got
that clear.

BOYNE: I've got it. Put your hand on mine. Keep your gaze
directed right here at me. Don't take your eyes from
mine. Take a deep breath now and fill up your lungs.
I'm going to count from five down to one. As I do,
your eyelids grow heavy, droopy, drowsy, and sleepy.
By the time I reach the count of one, they close right
down, and you go deep into hypnotic slumber. Five,
eyelids heavy, droopy, drowsy, and sleepy. Four, the
next time they blink that's hypnosis coming on you
then. Three, your heavy lids are ready to close. Two,
they begin closing, closing, closing, closing, closing,
closing, closing, closing, close them. Close them.
Close them. One, sleep and relax. (Gil snaps his fingers.) That's fine. Let every muscle and every nerve
grow loose and limp and relaxed. When I use the word
sleep, you now understand it's not the kind of sleep
that you sleep at night. I'm referring instead to a very
pleasant state of mental and physical relaxation that
you're experiencing this very moment. I want you
now to relax and continue going deeper until I squeeze
your hand again now.

All right now, I'm back to you (Gil squeezes Tyler's
hand) and I'm addressing you. There is a feeling that
you are aware of, and it's a feeling that has to do with
females. It's a feeling of fear, nervousness, tension,
anxiety, and I'm going to count to three. When I
count to three, I'm going to ask you a question. You
won't have to think about the answer. The answer will
come up from your deeper mind by spelling letter by
letter. One, two, three. What is it that causes you to
feel that feeling of fear, anxiety, nervousness, tension?
Just a word, quickly. Just the first letter. Speak.

TYLER: G.

BOYNE: The next.

TYLER: I.

BOYNE: The next.

TYLER: R.

BOYNE: The next.

TYLER: L.

BOYNE: The next.

TYLER: S.

BOYNE: All right. This time I'll tap your forehead. It will be a sentence, a phrase or a couple of sentences that use the word *girls*. (Gil taps Tyler's forehead.)

TYLER: Girls scare me.

INTENSIFYING THE PREDOMINANT SUBCONSCIOUS FEAR

BOYNE: "Girls scare me." I want you to become aware of that feeling of being scared as I count from one up to ten. It's a familiar feeling. One, two, three, it's a feeling of fear. It's a feeling that you'll be rejected. Four, it's a feeling that you feel of being unlovable, a fear, a feeling that you're not quite a man. Five, it's a fear of failing. Six, it's a fear of being ridiculed and laughed at. Seven, the feeling grows more and more intense. Eight, it's rolling across you now like a great wave. Nine, it's like a floodgate on the dam opening up. Number ten, I'm going to count from ten down to one. As I do, we're going back to an earlier time. A time that has to do with this very same kind of feeling. Ten, nine, eight, you're drifting back. Seven, six, five, you're growing younger now. Four, your arms and legs are shrinking and you're growing smaller. Three, two, one. (Gil presses on Tyler's head with his hand.) Where are you, indoors or outside? Make a choice quickly.

TYLER: In.

BOYNE: Daytime or nighttime?

TYLER: Night.

BOYNE: You're indoors. It's in the nighttime. Are you alone or is someone with you?

TYLER: Someone.

BOYNE: Who is it that's with you?

TYLER: Asha.

BOYNE: Asha is your girlfriend; is that right?

TYLER: Uh-huh.

BOYNE: You're indoors, it's in the nighttime, and you're with Asha. How old are you?

TYLER: Fifteen.

BOYNE: Fifteen years old, and what are you two doing?

TYLER: Fooling around.

BOYNE: You're fooling around. How do you feel?

TYLER: Excited.

BOYNE: "I feel excited." Where in your body do you seem to feel the excitement?

TYLER: My chest.

BOYNE: In your chest. Can you talk about it? Does it have to do with your breathing? Is it a pounding of your heart? What's happening?

TYLER: My heart.

BOYNE: Your heart. Describe the feeling in and around your heart in a symbolic way. "It feels like..." or "It feels as if..."

TYLER: Suffocating.

BOYNE: "I feel like I'm suffocating." I'm going to count now from ten down to one. As I do, we're going back to an earlier time that has to do with this feeling of suffocating. Ten, nine, eight, you're drifting back. Seven, six, five, you're growing younger now. Four, three, two, one. (Gil presses on Tyler's head and taps his forehead.) Where you are, are you indoors or outside? Quickly now, pick one. Make a choice. It's a feeling of not being able to breath, suffocating, breathless. (Gil taps Tyler's forehead.) Is it daytime or nightime? Just make a choice. Don't try to think about it. Pick one.

TYLER: Nothing.

BOYNE: Nothing. This time I'm going to count from one up to four and we'll go up to another time. One, two, three, four, being more aware. Are you indoors or outside? Quickly now.

TYLER: Nothing.

BOYNE: All right. Talk about nothing. Start out with nothing. Say, "Whenever I try to think, all I experience is nothing." Say that to me.

TYLER: Whenever I try to think, all I experience is nothing.

BOYNE: Now talk about that experience of nothing.

TYLER: Nothing. There's nothing, I don't know.

BOYNE: I want you to enter into that experience and here's what I'll have you do. Become the nothing. Say, "I'm nothing," and then continue. Describe what it's like to be nothing, the experience of it.

TYLER: I'm nothing, I'm not anybody to anybody.

BOYNE: "I'm not anybody to anybody." What part of the body does that feeling come from, "I'm not anybody to anybody"? Pick a part of the body that it comes from.

TYLER: My chest.

BOYNE: From the chest. Take your hand and put it over the place where that voice speaks, "I'm not anybody to anybody."

TYLER: (He places his hand on his chest near his heart.)

BOYNE: Is your hand over your heart?

TYLER: No.

BOYNE: No. Tell me exactly where it is.

TYLER: Right to the—it's more the lungs.

BOYNE: Now, be the lungs. Say, "I'm the lungs," and every time you are speaking to that other part and have the thought, "I'm nobody to anybody and..." put an ending on it. All right, begin. "I'm the lungs..."

TYLER: I'm scared.

BOYNE: Start out, "I'm the lungs..."

TYLER: I'm the lungs and I'm scared.

BOYNE: All right. Tell the head how the lungs behave when you feel that fear.

TYLER: (He takes deep breaths.)

BOYNE: "I need to take deep breaths when I feel that fear." "I need to take a deep breath." Is that it? Or, "I feel like I need to take a deep breath but can't."

TYLER: No.

BOYNE: What is it?

TYLER: Kind of gasping.

BOYNE: Gasping for breath. Now can you stay with that feeling, that feeling of gasping for breath?

TYLER: Yeah.

BOYNE: Track it a little bit now. Let's count it down once again and go from six down to one and go to an earlier time that has to do with that gasping. Six, five, just follow the feeling and let it float backward. Four, three, two, one. (Gil taps Tyler's hand right in the chest as he says) Gasping for breath. Where are you now? Quickly.

TYLER: On the playground.

BOYNE: On the playground. How old are you? Are you younger than six?

TYLER: No.

BOYNE: Younger than eight?

TYLER: No.

BOYNE: Younger than ten?

TYLER: Yes.

BOYNE: Are you ten years old, nine years old? Pick one.

TYLER: I think nine.

BOYNE: You're nine years old. What has happened to you? What's going on?

TYLER: I'm with some guys.

BOYNE: With some guys. What are you fellows doing? What are you boys doing?

TYLER: Making fun.

BOYNE: Of whom or what?

TYLER: My old girlfriend.

BOYNE: Your old girlfriend. How are you making fun of her?

TYLER: Whatever comes up.

BOYNE: Why do you want to make fun of her?

TYLER: Because they are.

BOYNE: How do you feel as you see them making fun of her?

TYLER: She's looking at me.

BOYNE: What do you think her look means? What do you think she's saying to you in that look?

TYLER: What are they doing to me?

BOYNE: How do you feel?

TYLER: Like shit.

BOYNE: Keep describing it. Tell me what feeling "like shit" means. Go into your body. What's the feeling in your body?

TYLER: Everything is falling to the bottom, my lungs, my heart.

BOYNE: It's all sinking.

TYLER: Sinking.

BOYNE: What was up high is now sinking; is that right?

TYLER: Uh-huh.

BOYNE: What would you like to say to that girl?

TYLER: I'm sorry.

BOYNE: All right. When I count to three, she'll be seated in the chair and you're seated out in the chair in front of her. I'm going to have you talk to her. Call her name. (Gil taps Tyler's forehead.)

TYLER: Lori.

BOYNE: Lori. Say, "Lori, I want to tell you my feelings."

TYLER: Lori, I want to tell you my feelings. I'm sorry.

BOYNE: Tell her what you're sorry for.

TYLER: For those guys. For me following along.

BOYNE: Just say, "You know, I'm sorry I just went along with things instead of trying to stop it." Is that what you mean? Or instead, maybe kicking up a fuss?

TYLER: Kicking up a fuss.

BOYNE: Can you tell her why? "I was afraid that they might laugh at me," or whatever was the reason. Maybe she'll understand. Tell her now.

TYLER: I can't.

BOYNE: What is it that keeps you from doing it?

TYLER: My heart's pounding too hard.

BOYNE: "My heart is pounding too hard." Now, change places. You're in the chair. You're Lori. Speak to Tyler. He says he's sorry that he went along with the boys making fun of you. Tell him how you feel.

TYLER/Lori: About to cry.

BOYNE: Say it again.

TYLER/Lori: I'm about to cry.

BOYNE: How do you call Tyler? Do you have a nickname for him?

TYLER/Lori: Ty or Tyler.

BOYNE: Say, "Ty, I'm about to cry just as I try to talk to you here."

TYLER/Lori: Ty, I'm about to cry.

BOYNE: Change again. Now be Ty. Answer Lori.

TYLER: I wanted to hold you.

BOYNE: Say it again.

TYLER: I wanted to hold you and kiss you.

BOYNE: Now be Lori. Ty said he wanted to hold you and kiss you. Talk to him.

TYLER: (as Lori) I wanted to. I couldn't figure out what you guys were doing.

BOYNE: What does Ty say? How does he answer? Do you care about Lori?

TYLER: I did.

BOYNE: You liked her. Tell her that.

TYLER: I like you.

BOYNE: Now be Lori. Do you care about Ty?

TYLER/Lori: Yeah.

BOYNE: Tell him that.

TYLER/Lori: I care about you.

BOYNE: Can you understand and forgive him for going along with the gang?

TYLER/Lori: I understand.

BOYNE: Tell him that. Be Ty. Lori says she understands. What's happening in your chest?

TYLER: It's still pounding.

BOYNE: Can you stay with that feeling in your chest?

TYLER: Uh-huh.

BOYNE: Let's track it back once again. This time I'll count from four down to one and let's slide right on back. Four, three, two, one. (Gil taps Tyler's hand, which is over his chest.) Are you indoors or outside?

TYLER: Indoors.

BOYNE: Daytime or nighttime?

TYLER: Day.

BOYNE: Are you alone or is someone with you?

TYLER: Whole bunch of people.

BOYNE: Who is it that is with you and around you?

TYLER: Michele.

BOYNE: Michele. How old are you?

TYLER: Five.

BOYNE: Five years old. What's happening? What's going on?

TYLER: Kissing her.

BOYNE: All right. And how old is Michele?

TYLER: Same.

BOYNE: Same, five. What do you think of all this kissing? Do you like it?

TYLER: I'm a big guy on campus.

BOYNE: Now you're five years old. What do you know about

kissing? Did your brother tell you something?

TYLER: Friends—I don't know.

BOYNE: How do you feel as you're kissing Michele?

TYLER: My heart's pounding.

BOYNE: Your heart's pounding. I'm going to tell you about that. You see, there is kind of an excitement in doing things that you feel are new to you or maybe you were told you shouldn't do, and especially doing things like kissing and touching girls. That's also exciting, and you feel excitement in your breathing. You could feel it in your chest. You could feel it in your legs, and you can feel it in your penis. Are you ever aware of feeling any funny feelings in your penis when you are with these girls?

TYLER: Nothing.

BOYNE: All right. Let's come up now. As I count from one up to seven, come up to a time when you're older that has to do with these same kind of feelings. One, two, three, growing older now. Four, five, six, seven. (Gil taps Tyler's hand, which is resting on his chest.) Are you indoors or outside?

TYLER: Indoors.

BOYNE: Daytime or nighttime?

TYLER: Daytime.

BOYNE: You are indoors. It's in the daytime. Are you alone or someone with you?

TYLER: Whole bunch of people.

BOYNE: A lot of people around you. How old are you?

TYLER: Fifth grade.

BOYNE: You're in the fifth grade. You're about ten or eleven years old; is that right?

TYLER: Uh-huh.

BOYNE: What's going on?

TYLER: School just let out.

BOYNE: School just let out. How do you feel?

TYLER: Scared.

BOYNE: What is it that is scaring you? Say to me, "I'm scared of..." or "I'm scared because..." or "I'm scared about..."

TYLER: Scared because everybody is waiting for Lori and I to kiss.

BOYNE: Do you kiss while they watch? Is that it? What does it mean, "Everybody is waiting for Lori and I to kiss"?

TYLER: Well, they wouldn't believe it.

BOYNE: You told them, but they wanted to see to believe it.

TYLER: They didn't believe we french-kissed.

BOYNE: They didn't believe you had french-kissed. So you told them you would do it while they watched; is that it?

TYLER: Kind of.

BOYNE: You wanted to show off a bit. Big man on campus.

TYLER: Uh-huh.

BOYNE: What's happening now?

TYLER: Our teacher sees us.

BOYNE: There's the teacher. How do you feel?

TYLER: Scared.

BOYNE: Where do you feel the fear?

TYLER: My heart.

BOYNE: In your heart. Were you kissing her when the teacher saw you?

TYLER: Uh-huh.

BOYNE: What do you think is going to happen?

TYLER: I don't know.

BOYNE: Going to get in trouble?

TYLER: Uh-huh.

BOYNE: It seems like every time you're around one of these girls, especially if you do things like kissing, you get upset or get in trouble. Is it the way it seems?

TYLER: I just want to be cool.

BOYNE: You just want to be cool. What does being cool mean to you?

TYLER: Do cool things that other people don't do.

BOYNE: Let me tell you something. In that situation I think cool means maybe doing things other people don't and not showing any excitement while you're doing it, like it's nothing to get excited over. It's no big deal; is that right? Is that what being cool means?

TYLER: Yeah.

BOYNE: But you know certain things produce excitement and now a teacher saw you and that's liable to cause trouble, isn't it?

TYLER: Uh-huh.

BOYNE: What kind of trouble do you think?

TYLER: I don't know.

BOYNE: When I count to four, we'll go ahead in time to a time with your finding out about the trouble. One, two, three, four. (Gil taps Tyler's forehead as he counts.) Where are you now?

TYLER: Principal's office.

BOYNE: Principal's office. What's going on?

TYLER: He's talking to us.

BOYNE: Is Lori there with you?

TYLER: Uh-huh.

BOYNE: When I tap your forehead become aware of what he's saying. (Gil taps Tyler's forehead three times.)

TYLER: Can't be doing this in school.

BOYNE: Can't be doing this in school. What else?

TYLER: Lori is crying really hard.

BOYNE: She must feel very embarrassed, don't you think?

TYLER: Yeah.

BOYNE: Girls generally cry when they are very embarrassed. Do you think that's why she's crying or do you think something else?

TYLER: I don't know.

BOYNE: Maybe she feels foolish. What do you think it is?

TYLER: She's embarrassed.

BOYNE: Embarrassed, sure. What do you think the principal's going to do as far as your parents are concerned? Is he going to call home, tell them about it, or what?

TYLER: (He shakes his head negatively.) I would be cool if he called home.

BOYNE: Say it again.

TYLER: Thought I'd be cool if he called home.

BOYNE: How would you be cool?

TYLER: My mom.

BOYNE: When I tap your forehead, move forward to being with your mom. (Gil taps Tyler's forehead four times.) Where are you now?

TYLER: With my mom.

BOYNE: What's going on?

TYLER: Much older.

BOYNE: You're much older. Talk about your mother. How do you feel?

TYLER: Feel weird.

BOYNE: Can you describe the feeling weird and where you experience the feeling.

TYLER: My heart's beating fast.

BOYNE: Heart's beating fast. What else?

TYLER: Talking to her about sex.

BOYNE: When I tap your forehead become aware of something that Mother said to you about sex. (Gil taps Tyler's forehead.)

TYLER: I can't believe young girls fool around this early.

BOYNE: "I can't believe that young girls fool around this early." Is that right?

TYLER: Not me.

BOYNE: Oh, can't believe you fool around that early. Is that right?

TYLER: Yeah.

BOYNE: Mother seems disappointed in your behavior?

TYLER: Yeah.

BOYNE: What feeling is she expressing?

TYLER: She's happy.

BOYNE: She's happy. There are all boys in your family; is that right?

TYLER: Yeah.

BOYNE: Four boys to fool around.

TYLER: Uh-huh.

BOYNE: How do you think it would be if she had any daughters? Would it be okay for them to fool around?

TYLER: No.

BOYNE: No. (Gil puts his hand on Tyler's head.) Let your mind grow clear. I'm going to count from one up to ten. Come up to this time and place. One, two, three, four, five, six, seven, eight, nine, ten. This is the month of June in 1985. You're a grown man now. You have had an opportunity to look back and see some of the thoughts and ideas that influenced this boy and how they affected him as he grew, especially the connection between being with a girl, kissing, doing all those things and feeling as if he can't breathe, feeling the excitement in his body but needing to feel cool, making sure he never showed his excitement, and the kind of thoughts that came from those feelings and how those thoughts affected him as he grew and how those same thoughts are affecting you even today.

Now here's what I want you to do. I'm going to have you use your adult reasoning mind. When I count to three this time and tap your forehead, I want you to look back at the experiences of that boy, especially in relation to that feeling in his chest, and especially when he was with girls. See how those feelings emerged, how he tried to be cool and not show his feelings and live up to a kind of image that his brother put upon him or even his mother or his father. How that affected his behavior as he grew and how it may be affecting you today. Now take as much time as you need to analyze it, and when you understand it and are ready to talk about it, just raise this hand up. (Gil demonstrates with Tyler's left hand.) Bring it up here like this. All right. Three, two, one. (Gil taps Tyler's forehead.) Look back now and analyze the experiences of that young boy. (Tyler moves his left hand and places it on his body.) All right. Tell me about it.

TYLER: I was just a little kid trying to be cool.

BOYNE: (Laughter)

TYLER: Doing what other people didn't get to do.

BOYNE: Yes.

TYLER: I don't give a shit about them but I couldn't show it.

BOYNE: You got in the habit of feeling excited and scared but feeling that you couldn't ever show it. How did that affect you where girls were concerned?

TYLER: I like girls.

BOYNE: Sure you do. It's natural to be attracted to females.

TYLER: But I'm scared of them.

BOYNE: You always get that feeling in your chest like you can't breathe, don't you?

TYLER: Yeah, I'm afraid I'll be turned down.

BOYNE: "Don't want to be turned down." Sure. Everyone hates to be rejected.

TYLER: Don't want them to make fun of me.

BOYNE: "Don't want them to make fun of you." They'll say, "What's wrong with you, Charlie, can't you get it up?" "Great big, strong, good-looking guy like you, what's wrong with you anyway?" That's awfully embarrassing to imagine that happening, isn't it?

TYLER: Yeah.

BOYNE: You've imagined that happening often, haven't you?

TYLER: Too often.

BOYNE: Too often. My friend, you can understand how a young child came to these conclusions by trying to figure out how it was and how he should be. You can understand how he came to behave that way, can't you?

TYLER: Yeah.

BOYNE: How old are you now?

TYLER: Twenty.

BOYNE: You're twenty years old. Do you think it's appropriate for a man like you to continue to act as if you were six or eleven or fifteen?

TYLER: No.

BOYNE: No. What are you going to do about it?

TYLER: I don't know. I'm scared.

BOYNE: You see, Tyler, you came to accept certain ideas. One thing was good and right and appropriate. Boys felt one way and girls felt another way. Maybe because much of your upbringing was with your good, strong mother in the home, you came to feel and sense women as authority figures. It seems like you give a lot of power to females now, especially in this fear that they may reject you. Did it ever occur to you that girls have just as much fear about been rejected as boys do? Maybe even more.

TYLER: Yeah.

BOYNE: You know girls are more concerned about their clothes and spend more time combing their hair and doing their nails so that boys will accept them and find them attractive.

TYLER: I know I should say yes.

BOYNE: So they make the decision. They say yes or they say no and then you're rejected.

TYLER: (He nods in agreement.)

BOYNE: I understand that you have been thinking that way, but I want to tell you something. It's just not that way. Sometimes a girl decides when she sees a fellow that she really likes him and she'd like to get to know him better, and maybe even become intimate with him at an appropriate later time, but for most girls that thought really isn't in their minds. You have to learn to deal with what emerges; that is, you deal with the feelings that develop even when you feel your fear. I'm going to give you a suggestion right now that the next time you're with a woman and you feel that little bit of fear that you say, "This may sound funny to you, but right now I feel scared."

TYLER: No! No!

BOYNE: Why not? What would prevent you from doing that?

TYLER: I don't want to give them the satisfaction.

BOYNE: "I don't want to give them the satisfaction." Finish it, "satisfaction of..."

TYLER: Knowing that I'm scared. That's the way my old girl-friend was.

BOYNE: What's the way your old girlfriend was?

TYLER: So pretty and she took advantage of me.

BOYNE: How did she do that, Tyler?

TYLER: She talked to other guys and didn't want me to talk to other girls.

BOYNE: She talked and kidded with other fellows, but she didn't want you to talk and kid with other girls; is that right?

TYLER: Yeah.

BOYNE: How did you feel about that?

TYLER: I just let it go by.

BOYNE: Seems to me that was kind of unfair, wasn't it? One-sided.

TYLER: Yeah.

BOYNE: Did you ever tell her that?

TYLER: Oh, yeah.

BOYNE: What was her response?

TYLER: "Bullshit."

BOYNE: Is that what she said to you, "That's bullshit"?

TYLER: Uh-huh. Everything was great at the first of the relationship.

BOYNE: And then what happened?

TYLER: She started to become bossy and wanted things her way.

BOYNE: She wanted things her way, and then?

TYLER: I went along.

BOYNE: Say it again.

TYLER: I went along with it.

BOYNE: Went along with it just like you went along with the fellows back there, remember?

TYLER: Yeah.

BOYNE: Easier to go along with things than to struggle against them, isn't it?

TYLER: Things like that.

BOYNE: What was the payoff to going along with it?

TYLER: She slept with me.

BOYNE: You kept getting your nooky, didn't you?

TYLER: (He nods in agreement.)

BOYNE: You were afraid if she cut you off, you couldn't find it anywhere else, weren't you?

TYLER: Uh-huh.

BOYNE: Well, I'm here to tell you, the world is full of females and their needs are just the same as the needs of the male—their need for love, acceptance, affection, and approval. That can be expressed in many, many ways, and you know that. All the way from holding hands, going to a movie together, enjoying a meal together, a dance together, to physical lovemaking. Many ways, such as just talking, exchanging ideas, seeing new things together, going to a concert together. They are all ways of sharing life through each other, aren't they?

TYLER: Uh-huh.

BOYNE: But you know you are at an age where your hormones are jumping, and those sexual feelings really seem overpowering at times, don't they?

TYLER: Yeah. But when I'm with a girl I don't feel them. It's like so **cool** down there I can't feel anything.

BOYNE: When you're with a girl, it just feels "cool" down there.

TYLER: (He nods agreement.)

BOYNE: Who or what do you think is inhibiting the circulation of blood down there. You know the penis doesn't have any bones in it. It's much like a sponge, and when certain nerve centers are excited, these veins and arteries dilate and open up and there is a surge of blood in these large spongy cells in the penis and you begin to get an erection. Now if that blood isn't flowing in there in that way, you don't get an erection.

TYLER: No.

BOYNE: Now what do you think? Who or what do you think is inhibiting the flow of blood into your penis?

TYLER: My heart pounding.

BOYNE: Your heart pounding as a sign of what?

TYLER: My feeling scared that it won't come up.

BOYNE: When you have an emotionalized picture that you'll fail, your brain and your nervous system only respond to the picture. That's why you know in the Old Testament Job said, "The things that I have feared have come upon me." Whatever we fear and worry about creates a blueprint for the subconscious mind, which instantly picks it up. When you have that fear and you have that image of failing and being rejected, that tells your subconscious mind to clamp down on those veins and arteries and inhibit the flow of blood. Were you ever aware of that before this moment?

TYLER: I knew what a person thought, how you feel—

BOYNE: Affected your body.

TYLER: Yeah.

BOYNE: You've heard people say, "Just the thought of it gives me goose flesh. Just the thought of it sends chills up and down my spine." When someone is afraid to do something, they often say, "He got cold feet." Well, those expressions come from the fact that when you're fearful of something, the flow of blood to your extremities, your hands and your feet, is diminished in the same way and the capillaries out there aren't nourished, and there is a drop in body temperature. Do you see how that works?

TYLER: Yeah.

BOYNE: You're going to have a much greater understanding of what you've done to yourself and how you've done it, and your subconscious mind is now open and highly responsive to the good and beneficial ideas that I'm about to give you. Tyler, you're now moving into a wonderfully pleasant state of hypnotic awareness, and as you do, you are realizing that you have the right to sexual happiness. You deserve sexual pleasure. You were born with an unlimited capacity for enjoyment and pleasure. You are now moving through old barriers of fear and resentment and your true sexuality is asserting itself again. You are learning to love yourself more with each passing day.

You like women, you enjoy the company of women, and you enjoy talking to women. It pleases you to be with a woman. You like yourself even when there are no women present. When you are with a woman who attracts you, you feel a pleasant excitement in your body. You enjoy both verbal and nonverbal communication with a woman. Women are aware that you like them, and they return the feeling to you. Women like you and enjoy your company. Certain women find you attractive and enjoy doing things with you. When you are in an intimate situation with a woman, you feel a wonderful excitement in your body and in your feelings. You reach out and make contact and as you do, you begin to develop an erection. You deserve sexual pleasure and other people deserve sexual pleasure too. You accept your individual pleasures and preferences in sex. You like yourself enough to easily ask your partner to satisfy your personal sexual needs. You now ask for what you want in lovemaking. You deserve all the pleasure you can get and so does your partner. You trust yourself and you go at your own rate of speed. You can play any role in sex that you want to. You assert your right of pleasure in lovemaking. Your worth as a male is never dependent on either pleasing or seducing women.

You are good enough to be loved by a woman. Women desire you sexually. You now practice being good to yourself. You can now attract a woman who is intelligent, warm, open, and affectionate. You accept women as they are. You have confidence in your lovemaking. You easily give yourself pleasure. You think of yourself as a winner. You constantly create new friends. You reward yourself and you never punish yourself. You nourish yourself with good food, enriching ideas, and nurturing friends. You are equal to any man. The more you love yourself, the more others love you. The more you love others, the more they love you. You constantly contribute to your feelings of aliveness and excitement.

You are passionately interested in people. You are a participant in life and you are loved for it. You are loving, generous, and expansive, and this comes naturally to you. You allow love to flow into your life and to flow out again when necessary. You allow people to love you. You accept the love, affection, and approval that others have for you. You attract loving people. You now forgive yourself for every mistake that you have ever made. You forgive everyone who has ever hurt you. Your true lover is being attracted to you now, for you are loving, you are lovable. You now draw to you friends and lovers you have been waiting for. You deserve love just for being alive. You can survive with a woman or without a woman. Your positive thought and action attracts positive and creative people into your life and they nourish you. The love inside you now flows outward in an easy, natural way. You are secure in a relationship with a woman. You now develop loving, harmonious relationships with women. You use each relationship for your own growth and expansion, and for the growth and expansion of your partner as well. You now know yourself better, and you communicate with others better than ever before. You are achieving self-awareness through being alone. You can be alone as much as you want to, and you can stop being alone any time you want to. You give your sexual partner freedom and she loves you for it. You approve of yourself whether you have a lover or you are celibate. You can be nourished and satisfied by one person, and you choose what is right for you. You allow others their freedom of choice.

You know that sexual loving with the right person is natural, normal, and healthy. You are an enjoyer and never a performer. You know that to perform means a performer and an audience, and you know that sexual loving is an experience shared by two persons. The more love you give, the more spiritual you become. You are powerfully interested in females. You are now fully aware of your desires. You are willing to express your sexual desires. You can be aroused by fantasies and you enjoy your fantasies and you learn from them. You love your body. You love your penis. You could enjoy being nude. You take good care of your body. Your body responds easily to sexual stimulation. You feel excitement in every part of your body. You develop a powerful, throbbing erection when you want to, and when you need to. You enjoy being a man. You are proud of your sexuality. You feel strong and sure as a man. You are free to frolic in pleasure. It is safe to let go as you approach orgasm. It helps you to experience ecstatic feelings more deeply. You can take all of the time that you need. You enjoy having an orgasm. You are willing to surrender.

You have the right to bring pleasure to your body. You enjoy touching others and being touched. You are warm and affectionate and you like making love. The more feeling you allow yourself, the more you can love and be loved. You reserve the right to say no to anything that you don't fully enjoy. You now forgive all women who have ever hurt you, and you can now let women love you. You find so much pleasure and satisfaction in loving you no longer care about getting even or feeling resentful. You are as naturally potent as you let yourself be. You are fully approved by your lover. You are free of fear and anger and resentment toward women. You are poised, charming, relaxed, and free with women to whom you are strongly attracted, especially in lovemaking. Your love and your self-esteem have overcome your old fears. You allow yourself to be overwhelmed with the total satisfaction of a powerful orgasm.

After intercourse you feel warm, intimate, and close to

your partner. You have the right to sexual happiness for you are a powerful, vigorous, potent man. You now realize that other women are not your mother and you don't need to act as if they were. You can now let women love you sexually as well as every other way. You are now rewarding yourself by fully, completely enjoying loving. You find so much pleasure and fulfillment in sex, you no longer care about controlling, getting even, or feeling resentful toward women. You fully approve of your own sexuality, and your body is for you to use creatively and enjoy fully. You now forgive your parents for withdrawing and withholding love from you when your behavior displeased them. You are now free of old childish attitudes about loving and about your own body. You now expel any negative attitudes about sexual loving that you held in the past. You now forgive yourself for not enjoying your body in the way you always wanted to and needed to. Each of these ideas has made a vivid, deep, permanent, mental impression in your subconscious mind, and each day in your daily life you become more and more aware of the full, powerful, positive, creative expression of these ideas.

I'm going to have you listen to these special ideas every day, and day by day you're going to find that the ideas most suitable for you will be accepted and you'll behave in ways that are fully in keeping with those ideas. However, if any ideas are not particularly appropriate for you in any given time, there is no need for you to accept them. You see, bit by bit and day by day and idea by idea, you will accept those ideas that will bring to you the fulfillment that God and nature intended for you to have. Now in just a moment I'm going to get you up. Before I do, is there anything further that you want to say to me, ask me, or tell me?

TYLER: I'm scared.

BOYNE: That's a familiar feeling. Now I'm going to tell you something. You use "scaring yourself" as a substititue for your natural erotic feelings. Are you aware of that?

TYLER: No.

BOYNE: I know that you don't want to, but that is all about to change. Very quickly, who do I remind you of?

TYLER: Teacher.

BOYNE: How am I like a teacher?

TYLER: Sharon Hayes.

BOYNE: Sharon Hayes. Is that a school teacher you had?

TYLER: Uh-huh.

BOYNE: Tell me about the qualities that I share with Sharon Hayes.

TYLER: Both brilliant.

BOYNE: Both brilliant. Did you have good feelings toward Sharon Hayes?

TYLER: Uh-huh.

BOYNE: Tell me how you felt about her.

TYLER: Mother.

BOYNE: She was like a mother to you. She was supportive?

TYLER: Uh-huh.

BOYNE: Helped you to learn and understand things.

TYLER: Uh-huh.

BOYNE: You knew you could depend on her and trust her.

TYLER: Uh-huh.

BOYNE: Are any of those the qualities that you experience in me?

TYLER: Uh-huh.

BOYNE: Wonderful. When I count from one to five, let your

eyelids open. You are calm, rested, refreshed, relaxed, and you feel good. One, slowly, calmly, easily, and gently returning to your full awareness once again. Two, each muscle and nerve in your body is loose and limp and relaxed. You feel good. Three, from head to toe you're feeling perfect in every way. On number four, your eyes begin to feel sparkling clear. On the next number now, eyelids open, fully aware, feeling wonderfully good. Number five, eyelids open now. Take a deep breath. Fill up your lungs and stretch. You really were in a deep trance today.

TYLER: (Chuckles)

BOYNE: Were you aware of how deeply you were in hypnosis today?

TYLER: I know I didn't have any eyes. The more you talked, it seemed, the darker it got.

BOYNE: (Laughter) I'm going to have you come in sometime and look at yourself here on the video. Any further comment before we close up? How do you feel?

TYLER: I feel good.

BOYNE: How's your chest?

TYLER: It's all right, it's not pounding.

BOYNE: Put your shoulders back and take a good deep breath and fill up your lungs.

TYLER: (He does as requested).

BOYNE: How does that feel?

TYLER: A lot better.

(BOYNE ADDRESSES THE AUDIENCE)

BOYNE: You begin to see the habituated response of the nervous system. Each time the nervous system responds in a given way, it becomes easier for it to react that way the next time, especially if it is accelerated by emotion such as fear. The fear of rejection is the most dominant fear in all of human existence because it strikes against our most powerful and deepest need—the need for love, acceptance, affection, and approval. Without some measure of satisfaction of those needs, we always remain dissatisfied and unfulfilled. The therapist has an opportunity to help the person to discover that they are indeed lovable. That the "unspeakable truth" they believed about themselves, *that they were unlovable*, is really just another perversion and distortion of reality. We must bring them to discover the reality of their true nature, "I am a lovable being."

Until the next time, this is Gil Boyne.

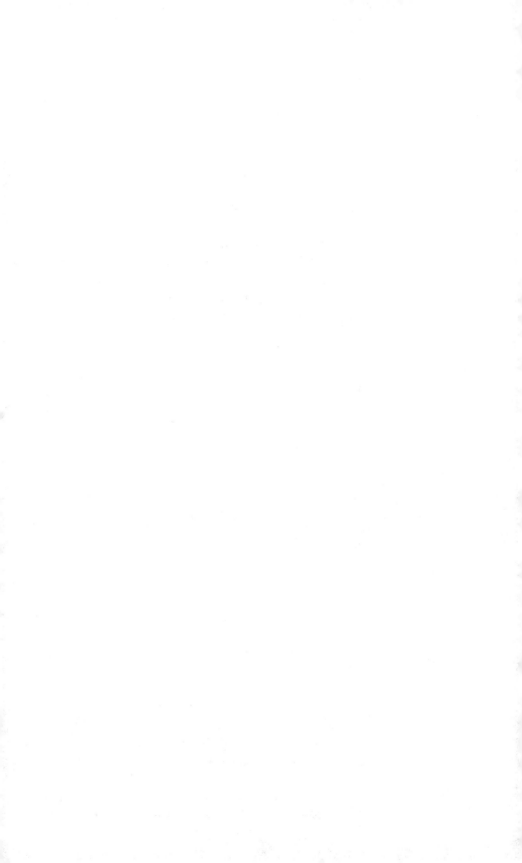

HYPNOTHERAPY TO CURE STUTTERING

The Case of Leo the San Diego Stutterer
("Please Don't Cut It Off!")

In two dramatic hypnotherapy sessions, Gil Boyne uncovers the "battered child" syndrome as an initial sensitizing event for a lifelong pattern of stuttering: a shocking conspiracy by mother and physician creates a castration trauma.

Age regression, Gestalt dialogues, bodywork techniques, and "Parts" therapy create an emotional transformation.

Three years later, Leo remains totally free of stuttering.

THE CASE OF LEO
THE SAN DIEGO STUTTERER
Please Don't Cut It Off!

(The Setting: A Classroom)

BOYNE: Hello. This is Gil Boyne, and welcome again to the Hypnotherapy Video Clinic. Today we're starting a new case history which was recorded live in San Diego, California, before ninety hypnotherapists.

INTRO: Gil Boyne is the only therapist I've ever seen or know of that works with clients he has never seen before and lets the chips fall where they may, and they always fall exactly in the right places. I am delighted to introduce the world's most effective hypnotherapist, Gil Boyne.

BOYNE: Thank you. Let's begin.

(BOYNE ADDRESSES LEO)

BOYNE: Tell me your first name, please.

LEO: Leo.

BOYNE: Leo, how can I help you today?

LEO: Well, I'm a little scared sitting up here.

BOYNE: That's to be expected—scared and kind of excited.

LEO: I—I had the idea for a while I would just walk out and not come back, which I almost did. And then I figured, I went this far so it c-c-can't hurt me, really, except you hate to be exposed in front of a b-b-bunch of people when you've been wearing a mask all your life.

BOYNE: Let me help you with that. We all develop a belief that if people came to know us, to see us as we see ourselves, or if we were to be fully revealed that they wouldn't like us. The boss would fire us, the wife would leave us, and so on. But the real truth is that revelation breeds intimacy. As we reveal ourselves, we become more intimate not only with those central figures closest to us, but with everyone. So you've gone past that state, and you're ready to begin. How can I help you today?

LEO: I stammered all my life, off and on, i-i-it goes up scale, down scale. Right now, I'm pretty much determined to handle it as best I can because I don't like people to see me stutter. When I do, I feel about this big. (Leo indicates with his thumb and index finger about an inch tall.) That's—I'd like to get r-r-rid of that if at all possible.

BOYNE: Do you make a difference between the word *stutter* and the word *stammer* and if you do, what's the difference?

LEO: I don't really make a difference between the two.

BOYNE: Many use them interchangeably. In speech therapy, stuttering is called a difficulty in beginning and stammering a difficulty in ending.

LEO: I suppose it would more be a d-d-difficulty in beginning.

BOYNE: All right. At what age do you recall this problem being present?

LEO: About eight.

BOYNE: Any other members of your family that had a similar problem?

LEO: Not to my knowledge.

BOYNE: Are you married?

LEO: I have been married. I am now divorced.

BOYNE: Did you have this speech inhibition in talking to your wife?

LEO: Sometimes.

BOYNE: Were those sometimes when you were angry, quarreling, upset?

LEO: If I'm angry, I don't stutter.

BOYNE: Have you ever had pets?

LEO: Yes. I've had a dog as a boy and had a horse as a boy, and we had a poodle when I was—I was married.

BOYNE: When you speak to your pets, do you stutter or stammer?

LEO: No.

BOYNE: All right. Now let's go the other way. What kind of a situation, circumstances, or people are likely to provoke stuttering and stammering?

LEO: Authority, and if I'm going to try to ex-x-plain something to somebody, I'll usually get a little uptight. It's as if I'm—I expected them to come back in some way. I'm not q-q-quite sure w-w-what that is.

BOYNE: Let me clear that up for you. That's a fear of criticism. You said, "If I'm expected to explain something and I'm expecting them to come back in some way." They're going to make an appraisal of what you said. That's the most common fear and everyone suffers from it to one degree or another. Because of the fear of criticism, the stutterer is constantly projecting outward their own negative feelings about themselves. You said a moment ago, "I feel that big." (Gil demonstrates with his thumb and index finger.) Stutterers rarely recognize that everyone stutters or stammers regularly. If you can pay attention to it, you'll find as I talk with you, even though I'm fluent most of the time, occasionally I will stutter, make a false start, back up and begin again; but I don't focus on it. To me, it's a part of my natural speaking rhythm and because I don't focus on it, I manage it easily.

LEO: Obviously.

BOYNE: Give me an example of some persons or some situation you consider where you're speaking to authority.

LEO: (He sighs deeply.) I used to walk in and I used to like to smoke Camels but if on a given day I couldn't say Camels, I'd ask for Pall Malls. I was constantly changing brands because just the s-s-switch over in saying the brand name might be easier.

BOYNE: How about ordering food in a restaurant? Did you ever change what you wanted to order because you felt you might stutter if you said what you wanted, fried fish or whatever?

LEO: T-t-there are times I may have avoided saying a word. I call that "word avoidance," I j-j-just go to some other word that's easier and i-i-it'll be great.

BOYNE: Have you made any efforts, either on your own or with professional guidance, to get some help ?

LEO: Yeah.

BOYNE: Tell me about those efforts.

LEO: Back while I was at the U-U-University of M-M-Michigan, I started speech therapy there with Dr. B-Bartelsmann. That's a long time ago. He had a theory about one side of the brain and the other side, so he had me change hands so now I can write with both hands and do everything with both hands, but it didn't do any good. And I did some work while I was at the University of W-W-Wyoming. I forget what their theory was down there.

BOYNE: (Laughter) Hard to recall the many, many theories that you were exposed to and paid for the experimental use of those theories and no refund if you don't get a result.

LEO: No, no guarantees. And I've done a couple of years of psycho-cho-therapy to see if th-th-they could get a line, positive factor, or whatever. That didn't seem t-t-to work.

BOYNE: Was that with a psychiatrist, psychologist?

LEO: That was with a psychiatrist.

BOYNE: Two years, and how often did you see him? What was the frequency of your visits?

LEO: Every week.

BOYNE: Once a week?

LEO: Uh-huh.

BOYNE: About a hundred sessions?

LEO: Something like that.

BOYNE: The cost per session.

LEO: I think at that time, he-he-he was one of th-th- the best in the area. I think he was $65 an hour at that time. That's a long time ab-b-bout fifteen years ago.

BOYNE: You spent about $6,500—a hundred sessions times sixty-five.

LEO: Oh, I think did—I'm-m sure I spent more than that, but anyway it didn't make any difference.

BOYNE: Can you tell me the benefit that you achieved for that expenditure of time, energy, and money?

LEO: Well, I-I usually felt better when I walked out, but all the old patterns always came back.

BOYNE: The effects were temporary and transient?

LEO: Yes.

BOYNE: Were there any other benefits outside of this area of speech inhibition that you got from the therapy?

LEO: Only the fact that I did feel better when I walked out than I did when I walked in, and I r-r-really didn't notice any change. I finally got disgusted and didn't go back.

BOYNE: You mentioned the speech therapy and the various theories. It's only been very recently that hypnotherapy has entered into the treatment of speech and communication disorders at the academic level. I remember a lady who came into my training program who was studying to be a speech pathologist. The training requires a Master's degree and a special curriculum to qualify for state licensing. This woman had read somewhere that hypnotherapy was very useful in helping stutterers, and she asked the professor at the university about it and he told her, "Absolutely not. Hypnosis couldn't be of any help." Each month a psychiatrist came in to teach the class, and she thought, "I'd just save the question for him." When he came in and she asked him, he became agitated and told her not to raise the question again, it had already been answered and that there was no possible use for hypnosis with stutterers. This lady said to me, "At that moment I became determined to study hypnotism. By the mere intensity of their negative response, I knew they were covering something up."

Since then we've had some major breakthroughs. Speech pathologist Dr. Kenneth Knepflar of Pasadena came to study with me, and he got the "hypnosis fever," and since then he's written many papers and developed a line of cassettes for speech and communication disorders. We are finally penetrating into that academic community and they're beginning to see the amazing results.

LEO: One other therapy I had for about t-t-two or three months w-w-when I was about eight or nine years old, my mother took me to a, what do you call these guys that hit you in the back of your head?

BOYNE: Chiropractor.

LEO: A chirop-p-practor and he said the bones weren't lined up there. I can still remember that when I get a stiff neck. In fact, I'm getting a stiff neck just thinking about it.

BOYNE: Put your foot on the floor. It might help your neck. (Leo uncrosses his legs.) Like most sufferers with a chronic problem who failed to get relief, you've sought help in a great variety of places.

LEO: Uh-huh.

BOYNE: You've been used as the subject of experimentation in an attempt to validate many theories, and you seem to feel that you haven't had very much help.

LEO: I think the most help I have had has been on my own, just imagining; and sometimes it works, but it doesn't s-s-stay there any length of time.

BOYNE: I'm not sure, I'd like you to repeat that again. You said, "Just imagining."

LEO: Just imagining speaking well. I was with a sales or-ganization for two years, and I-I-I hired a gal t-t-to give the pitch. This was in '79, back in land sales. Because I stuttered, I couldn't do it. I didn't t-t-tell the people who hired me that because I did cover it well enough when they hired me. One night she got mad at me, and she said, "The hell with this" and walked out. Now I had to do it. I got up—I've never been nervous in my life. Anyway, I went home and I taped it. I retaped it. I s-s-sound terrible on tape. I heard my G-G-German accent and the little stutters magnified.

BOYNE: Are you aware at this moment of the intense self-criticism that you're expressing? Continue. Now your eyes have become very moist. Tell me what you're feeling. Your jaw is trembling. Stay with that feeling. What's going on?

LEO: (He appears to be holding back tears.) Nothing.

BOYNE: Close your eyes and go inside and make contact with that feeling. Describe the feeling. Start with, "I feel."

LEO: (He wipes his eyes.) I'm pissed!

BOYNE: Stay with the feeling.

LEO: It's a feeling like you're going to lose control.

BOYNE: I'd like you to do one more thing. Instead of saying, *you're*, say, "like *I'm* going to lose control." Would you repeat it that way? "It's a feeling…"

LEO: Okay. It's a feeling like I'm going to lose c-c-control. I don't know where the tears come from. They just come sometimes. It pisses me off.

BOYNE: Close your eyes. I'm going to give you a stem or a beginning of a sentence, and I'd like you to put an ending on it. "If I ever really lose control…" Repeat that.

LEO: (He sighs deeply.) If I ever really lose control…

BOYNE: Finish it.

LEO: I may kill somebody.

BOYNE: True or false? Are you a potential murderer?

LEO: (He opens his eyes and says) I used to daydream about it. (Tears are running down his face.) Aw shit! (He rubs them away.)

BOYNE: Close your eyelids down, please. Can you enter into that feeling of anger and murderous rage, and start like this, "Every time I think about or every time I thought about…"

LEO: Every time I thought about, I-I-I don't know w-w-what you want m-m-me to finish this with.

BOYNE: Whatever comes to mind. Remember, you just said, "I used to think about it sometimes, that murderous feeling."

LEO: I used to daydream about, you know, n-n-not any special in-in-individual, just (He releases a deep sigh) oh, slaughtering loads of people for n-n-no reason at all. It was kind of dumb, but-t-t I guess it took some tension off, or something.

BOYNE: All right.

LEO: That goes back as far as I can remember.

BOYNE: Are you aware of feeling guilty about such thoughts or anxious or surprised or nervous that you held those kind of scenes in your mind?

LEO: N-N-Not especially, no.

BOYNE: No. All right. So even though you might have held those fantasies, you never felt that you might act them out?

LEO: No, I know I wouldn't act them out.

BOYNE: All right. You knew that you held the control.

LEO: Uh-huh.

BOYNE: Now let's go back and put a different ending on, "If I ever really lost control..." Say that again.

LEO: If I ever r-r-really lost con-con-control, I would be afraid of what I would do.

BOYNE: "I would be afraid of my own behavior—actions"?

LEO: Uh-huh, very much.

BOYNE: Start again. "If I ever really lost control..."

LEO: If I ever really lost control, I would be afraid of what might happen.

BOYNE: "I'd be afraid of what I might do," and how about the consequences?

LEO: I-I-I n-never thought about that too much.

BOYNE: It never enters into the picture?

LEO: No, because I know I never would.

BOYNE: All right. Begin once again. "If I ever lost control..."

LEO: If I ever lost control, I would (pause)—no, it's j-j-j-just the t-t-thoughts, no.

BOYNE: Allow yourself to have the thought, allow yourself to have the scene.

LEO: I guess I want to ask w-w-what feeling? I'm (pause)— I often feel like I don't feel.

BOYNE: Repeat after me. "I often feel out of touch with my feelings." Say that.

LEO: (Leo takes a deep breath.) I often feel out of touch with my feelings.

BOYNE: Because just here a moment ago a feeling welled up in you and was expressed, through your eyes, through your tears, through the trembling in your jaw and in your lips. That was a feeling, and you were aware of it, weren't you?

LEO: I wasn't aware of-of f-feeling anything. It's j-just that tears well up without a-a-any feeling behind them.

BOYNE: I hear you saying that there should be some kind of thought process, maybe like a movie that you can react to with a feeling, then you'll know were the feeling came from. Is that what you're saying?

LEO: Yeah. That sounds logical.

BOYNE: There are thoughts and images and levels of aware- ness. We know that they're there and we can call upon them and we can play that movie up on the screen. It can be a well-remembered scene—a vacation, a per- son, a terrible experience that stays in the memory— and then there are scenes that flow from another level of awareness—subconscious awareness. A good ex- ample of that is dreaming. You don't plan your dreams. You don't say, "All right, this is what I'm going to dream tonight and so on." Your dreams arise from a deeper level within you and take shape and form with a meaning and significance that usually is not easily perceived or understood. Do you agree to that?

LEO: Yes.

BOYNE: But dreaming is not the only way that these feelings and this imagery emerge. A nightmare, for example, is a dream in which such strong feeling is generated that it wakes you from your sleep and you become awake feeling frightened, and your heart pounds and you break out in a cold sweat. Certainly that's a strong feeling, isn't it?

LEO: Yes.

BOYNE: And it's coming from imagery, scenes? (Leo has his eyes closed all the while Gil is speaking.)

LEO: Uh-huh.

BOYNE: So it seems to be a rule then that a feeling follows an image, whether the image is held in our conscious awareness or out of conscious awareness or held at a subconscious level. Do you agree to that?

LEO: That makes sense.

BOYNE: I hear you saying that the feelings you experienced a few moments ago weren't emerging from your conscious awareness.

LEO: That's correct.

BOYNE: But they were emerging from your subconscious awareness, your feeling mind.

LEO: Okay. I can buy that.

BOYNE: The subconscious mind is called the feeling mind or the seat of the feelings. I'd like you to focus your awareness on the fact that ever since the feeling emerged until now, you've spoken very fluently and easily. Can you find any connection or does that link up with any similar experiences? You said a few moments back, "I don't stutter when I'm angry." Now you just experienced another strong feeling, and you haven't stuttered since.

LEO: I-I can't tie that together.

BOYNE: All right. The connection we're looking for is that quite often stutterers seem to feel, "Whenever I get emotional, I stutter," and that's not really the case. It's usually limited to certain kinds of imagery and the chief thing is "fear of criticism." You see, you gave away your eyes and you blind yourself because you don't see people out there as people. You see them as a motion picture screen, and you project your funny little movies out upon them. You're busy imagining that they think the same critical thoughts about you that you think about yourself.

LEO: (He nods in agreement.)

BOYNE: So you have no way of experiencing their response to you. You have written a script, directed it, produced it and are busy acting it, and writing the reviews all at one and the same time. True or false?

LEO: Yeah. That's an expectation, I guess.

BOYNE: That's a rotten thing to do to people; isn't it?

LEO: I'm not doing it to them.

BOYNE: What you're doing to them is you cut off your response from their wholesome reaction to you and ascribe to them the ideas that originated within you.

LEO: Okay.

BOYNE: That's a rotten thing to do to people, isn't it?

LEO: Never thought of it that way.

BOYNE: Think of it now. That's a rotten thing to do to people, isn't it? People want to be kind and caring and loving towards you and friendly. You just cut yourself off in

that self-centered way so that you have no real awareness of them, or all your awareness of them is colored
by those images you're projecting out into them.

LEO: Well, it's l-l-like if they r-really got to know me, they
w-w-wouldn't like me, so—

BOYNE: So what do you do to prevent them from knowing
you?

LEO: I guess, I'm-I'm (Leo takes a deep breath) I'm kind of
a-a-a loner.

BOYNE: "I alienate myself." Say that.

LEO: I alienate myself.

BOYNE: How do you do that?

LEO: I just d-d-don't make contact any more often that I—

BOYNE: Open your eyes. This is the world out there, so you
may look at an individual if you wish or none of them
or at the ceiling or whatever. I want you to make some
sentences to the world that go like this: "If you ever
really got to know me..." or maybe, "If you knew me
as I know myself..." and then put an ending on it.
Begin.

LEO: (He takes a deep breath and trys to hold back the
tears.) Where does that feeling come from?

BOYNE: We've already established that. (Leo is trying to control his tears by rubbing his eyes.) Speak now. "If you
ever really got to know me..." (Leo takes a very deep
breath.) Please begin.

LEO: (His eyes are very moist and he rubs the tears from
them.) Yeah.

BOYNE: I'm going to give you a secret now. The more you
struggle against the feeling, the more it's going to
overwhelm you. But if you just forget it, you'll be in
control of it. All right, now, begin. "If you ever really
got to know me as I know myself..."

LEO: If you ever really got t-t-to kn-n-now me, I have the f-feeling you wouldn't like me.

BOYNE: Start again.

LEO: If you ever really got to know me, I have the feeling you wouldn't like me.

BOYNE: Start again, put a new ending on it.

LEO: If you really ever got to know me...

BOYNE: What would they discover about you? You'd find out that...

LEO: (Tears are running down Leo's face.) I guess you'd find out I'm not such a bad guy after all. (He rubs the tears from his eyes.)

BOYNE: Say this one. Look out there, "If you ever really got to know me...'

LEO: (He sighs and tries to hold back his tears.) If you ever really got to know me...

BOYNE: "You'd find out how love-starved I am."

LEO: (He breaks down crying.)

BOYNE: What's the feeling? Tend to your breathing now. (Leo is sobbing.) Take some good, deep breaths.

LEO: (He is deep-breathing now.)

BOYNE: That's it.

LEO: (He breathes deeply again.)

BOYNE: Three, two, one. (Gil places his left hand on Leo's forehead as he says) SLEOP! Just go way down now, loosely, limply relaxing. (Gil is rocking Leo's head.) I'm going to count from ten down to one. As I do, we're going back to a time and place that has to do with this same feeling. (Gil taps Leo's forehead as he counts.) Ten, nine, eight, you're drifting back. Seven, six, five, you're growing younger now. Four, your arms and legs are shrinking, growing smaller. Three,

> two, one. (Gil places his left hand on the back of Leo's neck and gently moves it forward.) Where you are now, are you indoors or outside? Make a choice, quickly!

LEO: I'm inside.

BOYNE: Daytime or nighttime?

LEO: Daytime.

BOYNE: Are you alone or are others with you or around you?

LEO: I'm with my mother.

BOYNE: How old are you?

LEO: About six.

BOYNE: Six years old. It's daytime. You're indoors. You're with your mother, you're six years old. Give a report. What's going on?

LEO: I've got to give a poem.

BOYNE: All right.

LEO: A little t-talk on stage at the PTA (Parent-Teachers Association).

BOYNE: Okay.

LEO: And, and my m-m-mother, I have to know it p-p-perfectly a-a-and give it p-p-perfectly. (He tries to hold back tears.) So w-w-we're going over and over it again. She's v-very strict on ex-expression.

BOYNE: Mother's kind of a perfectionist?

LEO: Well, she—s-she used to teach d-dramatics before she got married.

BOYNE: I see. So you're six years old, and you're trying to please mother and get it down perfect. How do you feel?

LEO: I want to go out and play.

BOYNE: Let your mind grow clear. (As Gil says these words, he places his hand on Leo's forehead and rocks it a bit.) When I count to three, you'll be seated in the chair and your mother will be seated in the chair about six feet out in front of you. One, two, three. Now there sits your mother, and I want you to talk to her. And I want you to begin in this way—how do you address her? Mom? Mommy? Ma?

LEO: Mom.

BOYNE: Say, "Mom, I want to tell you my feelings." Start.

LEO: Mom, I'm going to tell you my feelings. I'm, I really don't want to get up on that stage. (His head is shaking from side to side as he's speaking.)

BOYNE: Tell her now you feel about it.

LEO: Well, last time I was there everybody laughed at me.

BOYNE: Say, "I'm afraid of being embarrassed and humiliated."

LEO: I'm afraid of being embarrassed and humiliated.

BOYNE: Now I want you to change places. Be the mother. Answer your son because he didn't want to get up on that stage and make that little talk.

LEO: (As the mother) But I want you to get on that stage so everybody can see what a bright little boy you are.

BOYNE: Be the boy.

LEO: I- (pause) I-I can't say it as well as she wanted me to.

BOYNE: Tell her how it makes you feel. "It makes me feel..."

LEO: (Tears are running down his face.) I guess I'm just kind of scared.

BOYNE: "Scared that you won't like me. You won't approve."

LEO: I'm scared you w-w-won't like me if I don't do it as perfect as you want.

BOYNE: All right. (Gil taps Leo's forehead as he says) Be the mother.

LEO: (As the mother) Well, I n-need you to be. (You can see the emotional pain on his face. He sighs deeply.)

BOYNE: Finish it. "I need you to be…"

LEO: (As the mother) I need you to be perfect. (He tries to hold back tears.)

BOYNE: Tell your son why you need him to be perfect.

LEO: (As the mother) I need you to be perfect so every—I guess s-s-s-so that people know that I'm p-perfect too.

BOYNE: Say this to your son. "I need you to be perfect because I have such an intense fear of criticism." Say that.

LEO: (As the mother) I need y-you to be perfect because I have such an intense f-fear of criticism.

BOYNE: (Gil taps Leo's forehead as he says) Be the boy.

LEO: Well, I'm afraid of your criticism.

BOYNE: Say it again.

LEO: (He begins to cry harder and sighs again.) I'm afraid of your criticism.

BOYNE: Again.

LEO: I'm afraid of your criticism.

BOYNE: Can you say, "I'm afraid I'll never please you."

LEO: I'm afraid I'll never please you.

BOYNE: Again.

LEO: I'm afraid I'll never please you.

BOYNE: True or false?

LEO: It's true.

BOYNE: (Gil taps Leo's forehead as he says) Be the mother.

LEO: (As the mother) You can please me if you'll try harder.

BOYNE: (Gil taps Leo's forehead and says) Now be the boy.

LEO: I d-do try hard, b-but I'm always a-afraid that when I'm, I'm s-saying the poem it won't come out right.

BOYNE: "I'm afraid that when I say the poem, it just won't come out right," and when it doesn't come out right, then what?

LEO: When it doesn't c-come out right, you s-scold me. We have to keep on going over it until it does.

BOYNE: (Gil places his hand on Leo's forehead and says) Let your mind grow clear. This time I'll tap your forehead and I want you to be the mother, and maybe you can explain to your son your attitude and perhaps how you came to be that way, maybe the way your parents related to you. Be the mother now and talk to your son. (Gil taps Leo's forehead.) "I'm this way because..." Maybe you could help him understand.

LEO: (As the mother) I'm this way because I was an orphan. (Leo starts crying.)

BOYNE: "Because I was an orphan." Tell him how the orphan felt.

LEO: (As the mother) I had to compete with the other kids.

BOYNE: "I had to compete with the other kids."

LEO: (As the mother) And I had to be-be perfect in the home in order to be liked. (Leo is wiping his eyes and nose.)

BOYNE: Can you say it to him this way: "I felt I had to be perfect in that orphan's home in order to be accepted"?

LEO: (As the mother) I felt I had to be perfect in the adopted home with the other kids around in order to be—to be liked.

BOYNE: (Gil taps Leo's forehead as he says) Be the boy. Tell her how you feel about her need for you to be perfect in order to be liked and loved.

LEO: Would you repeat that for me, please.

BOYNE: Tell her your feelings—she told you why she felt she had to be perfect as a child, and tell her how you feel about her putting that same feeling on you.

LEO: M-Mom, it's really difficult to s-s-satisfy you in-in saying that-that poem exactly the way you want it, and with all the ex-expression and everything else in it, it's just (pause). I want to please you. (He tries to hold back tears.)

BOYNE: "But I don't feel I can live up to your standards."

LEO: But I don't feel I can live up to your standards.

BOYNE: (Gil puts his hand on Leo's forehead and says) Let your mind grow clear. I'm going to count from one up to ten. Come up to this time and place. One, two, three, four, five, six, seven, eight, nine, ten. You're a grown man now. You see, perfectionism is a curse. It's one of the adaptations used by those who suffer from an intense fear of criticism. The rationale is, "If I do it perfectly, then I can't be criticized." Or in the child's case, the mother in effect was saying, "If the child does it perfectly, he can't be criticized and credit will come to me as his mother for helping him and training him. Approval will come to me—"look how well she trained him."

The problem is, the perfectionist is not one who's striving for excellence, but one who never gets any satisfaction. They're like a person climbing a mountain. As they get within fifty feet of the top, they have a mechanism that pushes the top up another hundred feet. So they're always climbing as opposed to someone who might climb the mountain, pull themselves up on the top, sit there and celebrate the fact. Even though they might think about climbing a higher peak next year, they feel proud and get satisfaction from what they've done. The perfectionist is never nourished by compliments and approval, and often hears criticism where none is intended. Can you identify with any of that either for yourself or for your mother?

LEO: Yes.

BOYNE: Tell me about it.

LEO: I—there w-w-were times in college when I wouldn't take the test because I was afraid I didn't know enough to get the "A's." So I'd take an incomplete and practically m-memorize the damn book so I could go back and get the "A" even though, everything I've done, even where I've suc-eeded very well, it was as if it was an accident.

BOYNE: For you success was always an accident.

LEO: Yeah. It w-was as if I r-r-really had nothing to do with it. I just happened to be there and lucked out.

BOYNE: Circumstance and good fortune conspired when you enjoyed a success?

LEO: Yeah. Like, if people really knew how—that it was only an accident, that they—

BOYNE: They'd know you really didn't deserve it.

LEO: Y-Yeah. I'd felt like a phony.

BOYNE: You've always felt like a phony. In almost every case the fear of criticism is the companion to what I call the "unspeakable truth" that we believe about ourselves, which is "I am unlovable." Then there's another part of that that we really don't like to look at, because if we really feel unlovable, we're also unloving, AREN'T YOU?

LEO: I put on a good act.

BOYNE: That's the phony part, isn't it?

LEO: Yeah. That's why I don't feel nothing. (He begins to cry.)

BOYNE: I don't believe you don't feel anything. I think that

you're afraid of your feelings and you constantly wage
a battle to avoid experiencing them. True or false?

LEO: Yeah. I guess that's true.

BOYNE: All human beings have feelings. It's the way we experience them or fail to that determines the kind of emotional life that we have. I hear you saying that your
emotional life is sterile and frozen, that your efforts
toward central relationships have been unsuccessful
and you continue to withdraw. We use our imagination to reassure ourselves that somewhere in the world
are the people, the circumstances, and the situations
that come together and enable us to fill our deepest
needs. When we lose that hope, life loses its meaning.
Then we have two alternatives. We can enter into
anti-life behavior or life-affirming behavior. The most
obvious anti-life act would be suicide, and that comes
in two forms—immediate suicide or slow suicide,
which means addictions: alcoholism, use of other
drugs, compulsive and indiscriminate sexuality, food
addictions, addiction to solitude. All of which are anti-
life behavior. Now, apparently, you're struggling
against reaching that place of despair. I have a question for you. You've been punishing yourself very
severely over a long period of time. At what point will
you know you've suffered enough?

LEO: I don't know.

BOYNE: Because I'm certain that you've experienced a great
deal of suffering for the lifestyle you've developed,
haven't you?

LEO: Yeah, I guess. I'm not happy.

BOYNE: You're not filling your deepest needs, the needs for
acceptance, approval, affection, love. It sounds more
to me like you're a bottomless pit. Nothing seems to
fill you up. You're stuck back there waiting for
mother's approval. After all, if your own mother can't

approve of you, then you must be a phony. You must not be worthwhile. You must really be unlovable. That's the way a child would reason, isn't it?

LEO: Yes.

BOYNE: I'm going to count from three down to one. I want you not to look back, but this time to do it differently. I want you to bring into focus your adult reasoning mind. I want you to look at that boy and look at his mother as well. I want you to see that relationship and how certain feelings developed in him and how those feelings created certain thoughts, and then how those thoughts and feelings affected him as he grew and how they affected him as a young man, and how those same thoughts and feelings are affecting you today. Look at it, analyze it, and a lot of understanding, awareness, and insight will come from it. When you are ready to talk about it, just lift your hand like this (Gil demonstrates by lifting Leo's right hand), and we'll talk further about it. All right. (Gil taps Leo's forehead as he counts) Three, two, one. Now look back and analyze the experiences of that boy.

LEO: I'm kind of a bad boy.

BOYNE: Say it again.

LEO: I'm kind of a bad boy.

BOYNE: "I'm kind of a bad boy." Why are you or how are you bad? What is it that you do that's bad?

LEO: Well, m-my mother tells me I'm bad.

BOYNE: All right. Do you love your mother?

LEO: I'm not sure.

BOYNE: What is it about your mother—what is it that she says or does or doesn't do that makes you unsure that you love her?

LEO: I guess because I don't know if she loves me.

BOYNE: What is it about her behavior that makes you uncertain that she loves you?

LEO: I get a scolding and she criticizes the way I talk. I guess s-s-she doesn't understand little boys.

BOYNE: Do you love your father?

LEO: No.

BOYNE: What is it about your father that makes you feel you don't love him?

LEO: (He shakes his head back and forth and begins to cry. He is also clenching his jaw.)

BOYNE: Clench it tightly, very tightly now. Stay with the feeling. Take a deep breath. What is it about your father that makes you feel this way?

LEO: I don't know.

BOYNE: What is it he does or doesn't do?

LEO: He beats me (hard crying).

(BOYNE ADDRESSES THE AUDIENCE)

BOYNE: Now you see the source of the unexpressed rage, that fantasy about slaughtering people.

(BOYNE ADDRESSES LEO)

When I count to three, I'm going to put you in that chair again. Your father's seated out in front of you. (Gil taps Leo's forehead as he counts) One, two, three. There's your father. There's your father. Speak to him. Say, "I want to tell you how I feel."

LEO: (He is crying.)

BOYNE: Speak to him now.

LEO: You big dummy, I'm just a little boy.

BOYNE: Say it again.

LEO: (He wipes his eyes.)

BOYNE: Say it again.

LEO: You're not supposed to criticize your father.

BOYNE: Don't tell me what you shouldn't do, do as I ask you to do. Speak to your father.

LEO: I-I-I think (He tries to hold back tears.)

BOYNE: Speak now.

LEO: He's an awful angry man.

BOYNE: Say, "You're awful angry."

LEO: You're an awful angry man, and I'm scared of you.

BOYNE: Say it again.

LEO: You're an awful angry man, and I'm scared of you.

BOYNE: Again.

LEO: You're an awful angry man, and I'm scared of you. (His voice is getting louder.)

BOYNE: Say, "You scare me."

LEO: You scare me.

BOYNE: Again.

LEO: You scare me.

BOYNE: Again.

LEO: You scare me.

BOYNE: Say, "I resent you."

LEO: I resent you.

BOYNE: "You scare me."

LEO: You scare me.

BOYNE: "I resent you."

LEO: I resent you.

BOYNE: Keep alternating.

LEO: You scare me. I resent you.

BOYNE: Louder.

LEO: I resent you.

BOYNE: Louder.

LEO: I resent you!

BOYNE: Louder.

LEO: YOU SCARE ME!

BOYNE: Louder. Louder.

LEO: (His voice is rising.) YOU SCARE ME! I RESENT YOU!

BOYNE: Louder.

LEO: YOU SCARE ME! I RESENT YOU!

BOYNE: Louder.

LEO: YOU SCARE ME! I RESENT YOU!

BOYNE: Louder.

LEO: YOU SCARE ME! I RESENT YOU!

BOYNE: Shout it.

LEO: (He screams it.) YOU SCARE ME! I RESENT YOU!

BOYNE: SHOUT IT!

LEO: YOU SCARE ME! (He is yelling.)

BOYNE: SCREAM IT!

LEO: (He screams it.) I RESENT YOU!

BOYNE: Again.

LEO: (Softly) You son of a bitch!

BOYNE: Go inside yourself and become aware of what you're feeling. What's the feeling?

LEO: T-T-The feeling must have blanked out again.

BOYNE: "I will leave the feeling." (Gil taps Leo's forehead.) Be the father. Answer your son.

LEO: (As the father) You're just a dumb kid.

BOYNE: Again.

LEO: You're just a dumb kid.

BOYNE: Again.

LEO: (As the father) And shut up and don't talk back to me.

BOYNE: Tell him that again.

LEO: (As the father) You're just a dumb kid. Shut up and don't talk back to me.

BOYNE: (Gil taps Leo's forehead.) Be the boy.

LEO: I will. (He grins.)

BOYNE: (Gil places his hand on Leo's forehead and rocks it and says) Let your mind grow clear. (Gil notices Leo's right hand is clenched into a fist.) All right. Let the right hand have a voice and speak to the head. (Gil taps Leo's forehead.) "I am the right hand." Speak.

LEO: I am the right hand.

BOYNE: Describe yourself, your nature, your form, your energy, size, usefulness, function. Begin. "I am the right hand."

LEO: I am the right hand. I am a boy and—I am the right hand. (He looks confused as he says he's the right hand.)

BOYNE: Be the right hand, and tell us all about yourself.

LEO: I am the right hand. I am the right hand. I think I'd like to smash something.

BOYNE: Say it again.

LEO: I'd like to smash something. I'd like to smash something.

BOYNE: Again.

LEO: I'd like to smash something. I'd like to smash something. (His voice is getting louder.)

BOYNE: (Gil places two pillows under Leo's right hand.) Raise your hand and bring it down.

LEO: I'D LIKE TO SMASH SOMETHING. (There is rage in his voice.)

BOYNE: Again.

LEO: I'd like to smash something.

BOYNE: Now say, "I'll kill you." Hit it.

LEO: (He starts punching the pillow.) I'd like to smash something.

BOYNE: "I'll kill you." Hit it. Say, "I'll kill you."

LEO: I'D LIKE TO KILL YOU, YOU SON OF A BITCH (angry and crying)!

BOYNE: Again. Again.

LEO: I'D LIKE TO SMASH YOU (with anger).

BOYNE: Louder.

LEO: I'd like to smash you.

BOYNE: Again.

LEO: I'd like to smash you.

BOYNE: Again.

LEO: I'd like to smash you.

BOYNE: (Gil is screaming) OPEN YOUR THROAT AND LET IT COME OUT. (Gil places his hand on Leo's throat as he says this.) Say it.

LEO: (He attempts to speak but nothing comes out.)

BOYNE: All right. Are you aware of how you lock your feelings and armor against your feelings by stiffening your muscles?

LEO: No.

BOYNE: All right. Let me help you with it. Armoring simply means the attempt to prevent the emergence of feeling. In this case here (Gil is holding Leo's arm with his left hand and with his right hand Gil brings Leo's hand up), this rigidity that you've created which moves up into here (Gil is moving his hand up Leo's arm to his shoulder and under his throat) and here and into the jaw line. Can you focus on that now and see how you do that? This is one of the ways that you cut yourself off from your feelings.

LEO: Like I'm holding back.

BOYNE: Many times today you've gritted your teeth as the feeling emerged, shook your head and restricted your breathing.

LEO: Uh-huh.

BOYNE: All right. Reverse the position of your hands. Just let them open up. (Gil is helping Leo open his hands.) Turn them a little bit. Open them up. Raise your arms. Hold them out and say, "Why won't you love me?"

LEO: (He shakes his head back and forth and tries to hold back the tears.) Why won't you love me?

BOYNE: Again. Say it.

LEO: No.

BOYNE: What's happening? Give a report.

LEO: I won't ask him—

BOYNE: Again.

LEO: I—

BOYNE: Open your chest (Gil puts his hand on Leo's chest.)

LEO: I won't ask him for anything.

BOYNE: Say it again. (Gil lightly strikes Leo's chest with his hand.)

LEO: I won't ask for anything.

BOYNE: Keep tightening. Tighten your legs. Tighten your entire body. Draw your knees up. (Gil is pulling Leo's knees up to Leo's chest.) Tighter. Tighter. Just pull yourself in. Say, "I won't ask anyone for anything."

LEO: I won't ask anyone for anything. (He has his knees pulled up to his chest with his arms around his knees.)

BOYNE: And that's just what you'll get, nothing. Pull your head down. Pull yourself up tighter, just as tight as you can. How does that feel?

LEO: Like I'm all squinched up.

BOYNE: When I count to three, let your legs drop to the floor. One, two, three. (Gil places his hand on Leo's head as counts.) Turn them all loose. (Leo's legs drop to the floor.) Tell me how it feels to release that restriction and tension.

LEO: Like I'm being exposed.

BOYNE: All right. Now that you're exposed, what kind of a feeling does that generate?

LEO: I guess I like the squinched up better.

BOYNE: All right. Do it.

LEO: (He puts his legs up to his chest and his arms around them.)

BOYNE: Draw tighter, tighter, tighter, every muscle. Tighten those fingers. Tighten the back of your neck. (Gil touches Leo's fingers and the back of Leo's neck.) Stiff. Rigid. Tighten your back. Pull yourself tighter. Become aware of the feeling. When I count to three, turn it all loose. One, two three. (Gil places his hand on Leo's forehead and says) Turn it loose. Now!

LEO: (He drops his legs to the floor and his arms to the side.)

BOYNE: Become aware of the feeling of being exposed. Any

other feelings that are linked with that exposed feeling?

LEO: I'm scared.

BOYNE: "I'm scared." Go into your body and tell me where you feel the feeling of being scared.

LEO: My genitals.

BOYNE: In your genitals. Describe the sensation. Is it a tingling, a burning, and itching, a vibrating?

LEO: No. Just like passing a gallstone—it hurts.

BOYNE: A feeling that you want to withdraw so you don't get hurt. Can you relate that to your sexual life? A feeling "I want to withdraw so I don't get hurt."

LEO: Uh-huh.·

BOYNE: Tell me about it.

LEO: Well I was about six years old. I was s-scratching my testicles because they had itched. They would stick together, and my mother kept scolding me, w-w-would spank my hands. She took me to the doctor and laid me on the table. They were going to cut it off. (He is crying loudly in a child's voice, very frightened.)

BOYNE: When I count from ten down to one, you're right back there on that table. Ten, nine, eight, seven, six, five, four, three, two, one. (Gil puts his hand on Leo's head.)

LEO: (Agonized cry) Oh, God, don't (terrified).

BOYNE: What's happening?

LEO: He's got a knife in his hand.

BOYNE: What are they going to do about it?

LEO: I don't know.

BOYNE: Why are you there?

LEO: Because I touched it.

BOYNE: You touched it. How do you feel?

LEO: I'm scared.

BOYNE: When I touch your forehead, you hear someone speaking, saying something either to you or about you. (Gil is tapping Leo's forehead.) What is it? What are they saying?

LEO: They're going to take care of it.

BOYNE: (He places his hand on Leo's forehead.) Let your mind grow clear. What your mother and the doctor are doing is very, very wrong. It's an effort to scare you into a form of behavior that they think is better for you, but it really is a great mistake, and it's natural for you to be frightened in this situation. But they're wrong. It's a very stupid mistake that they're making. When you grow up, you're going to realize what a mistake they made. When I count from one up to ten, come back. (Gil taps Leo's forehead as he counts.) One, two, three, four, five, six, seven, eight, nine, ten.

I want you to tell me now how you experienced that boy and that feeling "I want to withdraw so I don't get hurt," and a feeling of sexual excitement in your body, how they're bound together and how they affect you. When I tap your forehead, you'll recall a phrase, an idea will come instantly to your mind. (Gil taps Leo's forehead.) What is it? Speak now.

LEO: Bad.

BOYNE: "It must be bad." "God punishes dirty little boys," Mother says. You know it must be bad.

LEO: Yes, I-I just catch hell back then, you know.

BOYNE: Sure. Might even go to hell and burn.

LEO: (He in nods agreement.)

BOYNE: All right. Now come back up to this place with me. (Gil lightly taps Leo's forehead.) Become aware of a change in feeling of being open and exposed. Is there a difference in the feeling?

LEO: Yeah. I'm not quite as scared. I feel more relaxed like—

BOYNE: Can you say, "I'm beginning to relax"?

LEO: Yeah. I'm beginning to relax.

BOYNE: It's a nice feeling. Now be aware of being exposed in a number of ways, about revealing yourself and your legs and thighs are open, and in a certain way your genitals are exposed.

LEO: Yeah.

BOYNE: But it's okay because you are clothed?

LEO: Uh-huh.

BOYNE: And it's appropriate. Let's see if you can relate to a doctor or anyone else you want to put there as an authority figure. One, two, three. (Gil taps Leo's forehead.) Here's what I want you to say to them. If you're addressing Mother, you call her Mom or Dad or all of you or whatever it is. Who do you want to speak to first?

LEO: The stupid doctor.

BOYNE: All right. Tell the doctor.

LEO: He's really a dumb bastard.

BOYNE: Tell him that, "I think you're really a..."

LEO: I think you're really a dumb bastard.

BOYNE: Tell him why.

LEO: Little boys just scratch their penis. It's perfectly normal.

BOYNE: All right.

LEO: There isn't anything wrong with it.

BOYNE: Ask him how he could enter into such an arrangement with your mother to scare you that way.

LEO: How can you enter into such an arrangement with my m-m-mother to scare me so I, I won't touch it anymore?

BOYNE: (Gil taps Leo's forehead as he says) Be the doctor.

LEO: (As the doctor) Well, that's j-just a nasty, nasty thing to do and your own mother didn't want you to touch it, so we decided to just scare you into leaving it alone to make your mother happy.

BOYNE: All right. Now you're a grown man. You're not a helpless child anymore. Tell what you think of the whole process (Gil taps Leo's forehead) and finish it off. Close it down with a good statement.

LEO: Doctor Barton, you are a-a-a, one of the dumbest assholes I know. You really are.

BOYNE: Good. Now who else do you want to speak to that's over there standing out in front of you and seated in front of you?

LEO: My mother was, God bless her, r-r-really a warm, loving person. She didn't know how (His eyes are becoming moist) she had wronged me.

BOYNE: How are you like your mother?

LEO: I-I guess I'm the same in that she had to be perfect. She had the need to talk perfect, and she had the need for her kids to talk perfect and wanted them on the stage because that was the image of herself up there.

BOYNE: There she sits. Talk to her now. Tell her about this new level of understanding.

LEO: Mom, I understand that-that you're doing your best to make me into what you wanted me to be without knowing that you can't.

BOYNE: Can you say to her, "I now know that you were doing what you thought was best for me"?

LEO: Uh-huh. I know you were doing what you thought was best for me. I-I know that. I just wish you could have told me you loved me. (He begins to sob.)

BOYNE: Can you tell your mother that you love her?

LEO: (He tries to fight the tears.)

BOYNE: Now that you understand her, can you say that to her?

LEO: Mom, I want to tell you that I love you.

BOYNE: (Gil taps Leo's forehead and says) Be the mother. Answer your son.

LEO: (As the mother) Well, of course I love you.

BOYNE: Say it again.

LEO: (As the mother) I love you with all my heart.

BOYNE: Again.

LEO: I did the best things for you that I knew how.

BOYNE: (Gil taps Leo's forehead and says) Be the boy.

LEO: (Sharply) Well, you sure as hell didn't know how.

BOYNE: (Gil taps Leo's forehead and says) Now be the man.

LEO: M-M-Mom, I can understand where you were coming from, and it's okay because I can handle it from now on.

BOYNE: Say that again.

LEO: (Leo sighs deeply. Tears are running down his face.) Mom, it's okay what you did. I really do understand.

BOYNE: As you say that, I want you to feel that warm, pleasant feeling way down here expanding, starting to radiate outward. Say, "It's okay." Let it radiate into your genitals and upward into your chest. Say it once again.

LEO: Mom-Mom, it's okay what you did. It's okay. It really

is.

BOYNE: There sits your father. Talk to him!

LEO: You never listened to me before. I'm not so sure you're going to listen to me now.

BOYNE: "You're hard to talk to. You never listened to me before when I was a child, and I'm not so sure you're going to listen to me now." (Gil taps Leo's forehead and says) Be the father.

LEO: (As the father) Well, I-I was beaten as a little boy and that's probably why I beat you. And my father didn't have time for me, and that's why I never had time for you. And he never told me he loved me, so I can't tell you either. (Leo is sobbing hard at this point.)

BOYNE: Say to your son, "We learn to love by being loved, and I never learned that I was loved." Say that.

LEO: (As the father) We learn to love by being loved, and I guess my problem was that I didn't know how. I couldn't tell you I loved you, I didn't (sobbing).

BOYNE: (Gil taps Leo's forehead and says) Be the man speaking to his father again. Father says he never learned how. He just didn't know how.

LEO: Yeah. I know, Dad. They ought to teach it some place, and I guess now I'm sorry I, I waited until you died.

BOYNE: Say it again.

LEO: (Tears are running down his face.) I think I'm sorry.

BOYNE: Can you tell your father you love him?

LEO: No.

BOYNE: Find another word then.

LEO: (He struggles to hold back the tears.) Dad, I, I think I can just let it be.

BOYNE: All right. Is there anyone else standing there you need to talk to?

LEO: No, just two sisters there.

BOYNE: Anything you need to say to them?

LEO: No, except that I-I love them.

BOYNE: All right. Tell them. Call their names and tell them that.

LEO: Elaine, I-I do love you, y-y-you're my sister. Georgia, I love you too.

BOYNE: Repeat after me. "I now forgive everyone who has ever harmed me in any way."

LEO: I now forgive anyone who has ever harmed me in any way.

BOYNE: "I bless them with my love."

LEO: I bless them with my love.

BOYNE: "I want for them the same good that I want for myself."

LEO: I want for them the same good I want for myself.

BOYNE: "I forgive myself for every mistake that I have ever made."

LEO: (He sighs.) I forgive myself for every mistake that I've ever made.

BOYNE: "I now know that each mistake has simply been a stepping stone to greater understanding."

LEO: I now know that each mistake was merely a stepping stone to greater understanding.

BOYNE: "And to greater opportunity."

LEO: And to greater opportunity.

BOYNE: "I freely forgive as I would be forgiven."

LEO: I freely forgive as I would be forgiven.

BOYNE: How does that feel?

LEO: Kind of nice.

BOYNE: Go into your stomach, go into your chest, go into your genitals, into your thighs, tell me what you're experiencing.

LEO: My ulcer isn't bothering me.

BOYNE: Ulcer isn't bothering you. That's what's not bothering you. Tell me what you're experiencing—

LEO: Kind of a loose feeling.

BOYNE: "I feel loose." Anything else you want to report?

LEO: Yeah. Kind of like it isn't as dark.

BOYNE: I'm beginning to see the light.

LEO: (Laughter.)

BOYNE: That's how the song goes, doesn't it. (Gil takes hold of Leo's right hand.) There's a lot of reasons why we cling to old childish patterns. Sometimes I've discovered stutterers use their stuttering as a form of defiance.

LEO: Uh-huh.

BOYNE: A form of expressing anger that they feel they can't express in other ways, but they're the devices of the child. Now those things happened when the child was six and seven and eight and nine and ten. You can understand how the boy felt that way, can't you?

LEO: Uh-huh.

BOYNE: How old are you now?

LEO: I'm fifty-eight.

BOYNE: Fifty-eight. Do you think it appropriate that a fifty-eight-year-old man continue to behave and to act in life as if he were six or eight or ten?

LEO: No.

BOYNE: What are you going to do about that?

LEO: I am going to behave like a fifty-eight-year-old.

BOYNE: (Laughter.)

LEO: No, more like forty.

BOYNE: All right. (Laughter from the audience.) When you are able to, be like forty.

LEO: (He takes a deep breath.)

BOYNE: Now you can stutter or stammer whenever you want to, and you can speak fluently whenever you want to, and you demonstrated that here. You have no more excuses because you're here in front of ninety people, if anything would create tension and nervousness and anxiety, this would. And yet, you've spoken fluently and clearly for the last forty minutes. Are you ready to get rid of the defense patterns of the six-year-old boy?

LEO: You're damned right.

BOYNE: Repeat after me. "I am free."

LEO: I am free.

BOYNE: Make some statements about that now.

LEO: I am free means I don't have to, I can be me and if you can accept that, I can.

BOYNE: All right. Now open your eyes.

LEO: (He opens his eyes.)

BOYNE: Open them up. Look out at the world, and say this to them: "I don't have to live up to your expectations of me."

LEO: I don't have to live up to your expectations of me.

BOYNE: And that means—Tell them what it means.

LEO: It just means I can just be me and if you like that, that's fine. We'll get along, and if you don't, that's your problem, not mine.

AUDIENCE: (They applaud.)

LEO: I knew that intellectually all along.

BOYNE: Say to them, "And I now realize that you don't have to live up to what I've been expecting of you."

LEO: I realize that you don't have to live up to what I've been expecting of you, and that's like you had to show me some love before I could even c-c-come toward you.

BOYNE: Look at them and say this.

LEO: (Tears begin to flow.) I'm a damned loser.

BOYNE: Look at them. "For I am I and you are you."

LEO: For I am I and you are you.

BOYNE: And that means—

LEO: And that means I'm free.

BOYNE: Look at them and say, "From now on I'll do my thing."

LEO: (Smiling) And from now on I'll do my thing.

BOYNE: And that means—

LEO: And that means you can do yours.

BOYNE: (Laughter.) That's good. Going to let them do their thing even if you don't like it.

LEO: Right. Right.

BOYNE: So you can have the freedom to do your thing even though someone might not like it.

LEO: That's okay.

BOYNE: All right. Now look at them. Here's the punch line. Ready.

LEO: (He looks at audience.) I'm ready.

BOYNE: "If we can discover each other and have a loving relationship, it will be wonderful."

LEO: If we can discover each other and have a loving relationship, it would be wonderful. Yeah, it really would.

BOYNE: "But if that just can't be, I can accept that too."

LEO: If for any one of you that just can't be, I can accept that too. Yeah, I'm hysterical. (Laughter. Leo reaches over and hugs Gil.)

AUDIENCE: (They applaud.)

BOYNE: Put your hand in mine.

LEO: By the way, I had never hugged a man in my life.

BOYNE: Well, you just did. Look at me. Take a deep breath. Exhale. Just sleep and relax.

LEO: (His head falls forward.)

BOYNE: That's good. Now very quickly before I finish this portion of the session, is there anything further that you want to say to me, ask me, or tell me?

LEO: No, except I think I can let the past be the past.

BOYNE: All right. Let the dead bury the dead.

LEO: Yeah. That's history.

BOYNE: All right. Quickly, who do I remind you of?

LEO: Well, at the start you reminded me of my father. Right now, you're Gil Boyne.

BOYNE: What qualities do I share with your father?

LEO: Well, you're both strong men.

BOYNE: Strength. That's good. When I count from one up to five, let your eyelids open. You're calm, rested, refreshed, relaxed, and you feel good. One, slowly, calmly, easily, and gently returning to your full awareness once again. Two, each muscle and nerve in your body is loose and limp and relaxed. You feel good. Three, from head to toe, you're feeling perfect in every way. On number four, your eyes begin to feel sparkling clear. On the next number now, eyelids open, fully aware, feeling wonderfully good (Leo opens his eyes), light and free like a weight is coming off your shoulders, a rock has gone from your stomach, and you can feel any sensation in your genitals that you allow yourself to feel any time you want to, is that agreeable to you?

LEO: Absolutely.

BOYNE: All right. Wonderful.

(BOYNE ADDRESSES AUDIENCE)

Show your appreciation for this man.

AUDIENCE: (They applaud.)

(BOYNE ADDRESSES LEO)

BOYNE: Leo, what's your feeling toward this group now that you've revealed yourself to them?

LEO: I just feel warmth which I didn't feel before. Before you were a cold, sterile bunch of people out there. Now you're all real people. Yeah, it's warmth.

BOYNE: Leo's answer is warmth. When you deal with abstractions such as love, it's very difficult to find words that penetrate through their abstract nature.

I want to thank you for sharing with us and having the courage to do that, and I feel I've just been on an emotional roller coaster with you, and I think a lot of people feel the same way. It's really exciting what's happened, and I can see the joy coming from you.

LEO: Thank you.

BOYNE: (Laughter) This is the beginning of a happy New Year and a beginning of a happy part of your life. Leo, I want to thank you. (Leo and Gil shake hands and stand up.)

LEO: Thank you.

BOYNE: And I'm very glad that I reminded you of your father and his strength (Gil and Leo are hugging) because I know that you did have a lot of loving feelings for him. My father too was one who beat me regularly. He was a little man who got drunk every weekend and fought in barrooms to demonstrate something. I identified with what you had to say. My story was a little bit different in that at age sixteen I fought back, beat him up, and walked out.

LEO: I couldn't do that. He was dead.

BOYNE: If you get to work with some other hypnotherapist at some future time, not about the speech inhibition because I'm sure you won't need that, but there's a process called "saying good-bye." If I had more time to work with you today that's the next step I would take. You have a lot of friends now and they'll be talking to you.

(GIL ADDRESSES AUDIENCE)

Once again, show your appreciation to Leo.

AUDIENCE: (They applaud.)

BOYNE: This has been a good workaday kind of hypnotherapy. I hope that as you watch this film that you'll see a kind of road map. Remember, the subconscious mind is the feeling mind. When the client experiences feeling, the subconscious mind is open. Don't be concerned about trivial things as, "What kind of an induction shall I use?" Focus instead upon the elements of the problem and remember it's not really that complex. Once you clear your mind and liberate yourself from the many unproven theories about human behavior, you'll instead come to realize that we have basic needs and out of those needs come a fear that they won't be satisfied. You see, the fear of being unlovable, the fear of criticism, the fear of sickness and aging, the fear of death, the fear of poverty create the fear that we won't meet our essential needs.

Those of you that are acquainted with me know that I have had intensive study in many of the major psychotherapeutic systems, and I believe that my effectiveness in working comes because I have merged certain key elements from those systems into my therapies. In this particular demonstration you saw the use of Gestalt dialogues. I touched briefly into some of the principles of Bio-Energetic Analysis and the armoring of the body. You can be eclectic—take what you can where you can and merge it into a simple, workable process.

The client's needs are the same as your needs, for you're both human beings. Always deal with what emerges and listen to what they have to say. Don't have a road map for them and don't decide where they need to go. Let them walk with you and take their hand as they walk along and then later you can stand along side the road and say, "You're doing great. Just keep walking. Put one foot in front of the other." After you see they're walking well, you can turn and walk away because they're going to walk off and experience a life that has moments of being rich and full and free and satisfying. I'm especially pleased to be here with you, and for the time I've spent with you this weekend. I'm pleased because this is the fulfillment stage of part of a lifelong dream that I've had, and I thank God and the good friends that have been instrumental in bringing me to this point in recognition of my potential and the realization of the dream that began many years ago.

Until I see you again, this is Gil Boyne.

Postscript:

Leo entered into hypnotherapy and after three sessions he was totally free of stuttering. Later I watched a two-hour videotape of Leo's therapy, and he never stuttered. In the final segment of the tape he talked socially with ease with several class members and was fluent and confident. Leo was transformed!

Part Three

The Techniques of Transforming Therapy:

An Overview

PRE-INDUCTION, GOAL SETTING, UNCOVERING TECHNIQUES, AND AGE REGRESSION

Pre-Induction Interview

Therapist: Have you ever been hypnotized?

Have you ever made an effort to be hypnotized?

Was that for therapeutic purposes or for entertainment in a nightclub or theater?

Tell me about it.

Goal Setting

Therapist: If you were free of this (symptom, problem), how would your life be different?

Tell me what you want and need from me. Not what you don't want or no longer want—these are amputations. The goal is to be transformed, to replace the way you feel and experience life today with a new and better way. Tell me what you want to bring into your life!

Follow-Up Hypnotherapy Sessions

(Start session with this statement.)

Therapist: Tell me about your thoughts and feelings since our last session.

Uncovering Techniques: Intensifying the Underlying Feeling After Trance Induction

Therapist: There's a feeling that you hold about yourself. It's a feeling that you _____ (are unlovable, etc.). It causes you to feel _____ (anxious, fearful, etc.).

As I count from one up to ten, I want you to become aware of that feeling. I will grow more intense as I count.

One, two, three. Now the feeling begins to emerge.

Four, five. It's a feeling that you _____ (no one loves you).

Six. This feeling grows more and more intense.

Seven. You feel alone and unloved (etc.).

Eight. You feel fearful, nervous, anxious, afraid!

Nine. It's like the floodgates on a dam opening up and a great wave of feeling is rolling across you now.

Number ten. I'll count to three and tap your forehead, and I'm going to ask you a question. The answer will come out by spelling letter by letter. The answer will come up from your subconscious mind.

One, two, three. (TAPPING FOREHEAD.)

What is it that causes you to feel _____? (that makes you [eat, drink, etc.] obsessively?) The first letter, quickly. Speak out. (TAPPING FOREHEAD.) The next letter? (Etc.)

(After a word or words have been spelled out:)

I'm going to tap your forehead again and you'll speak a sentence, a phrase, or a paragraph that uses the word (*spelled word*). Speak. Now. (TAP FOREHEAD.)

Hypnotherapy: Age Regression to the Sensitizing Event

Therapist: I'm going to count from ten down to one. As I do, we're going back to a time and place that has to do with this very same feeling. (TAP FOREHEAD WHEN COUNTING.)

Ten, nine, eight. You're drifting back.

Seven, six, five. You're growing younger now.

Four. Your arms and legs are shrinking, growing smaller.

Three, two, one.

Where are you now, indoors or outside? Make a choice quickly!

Is it daytime or nighttime?

Are you alone or are others with you or around you?

How old do you feel?

You're _____ years old. You're (in/out)doors. It's (day/night)time and you are (alone/with _____). Give a report of whatever you see, hear, feel, or experience.

(WHEN THE SCENE HAS BEEN FULLY EXPLORED:)

Let your mind grow clear.

I'll count from one to four and when I do, you go to another time that has to do with this same feeling, a feeling of _____.

(OR, SIMPLY:)

Go to another time when you had these same feelings.

One, two, three, four. Where are you now, indoors or out? (Etc.)

SPECIFIC TECHNIQUES USED TO ELICIT INFORMATION

Examining Central Relationships (While Client Is in Trance)

Therapist: Do you love your (mother/father)?

Client: I don't know.

Therapist: What is it about your (mother/father)—what is it that (she/he) says or does or doesn't do that makes you unsure whether you love (her/him)?

Therapist: Does your (mother/father) love you?

Client: No.

Therapist: What is it about (her/his) behavior that makes you think (she/he) doesn't love you?

Discovering Scripts and Fixed Ideas

Client: They're shouting at me (...at each other).

Therapist: When I tap your forehead, you'll hear what they are shouting.

Discovering Sources of Fear (People, Places, Situations)

Client: I feel frightened.

Therapist: Make that a longer statement: "I feel frightened when..." or "I feel frightened because..."

Separate Person From Feelings and Behavior

Client: I'm so stupid!

Therapist: Can you say, "I act and feel as if I were stupid"?

Client: I must be strong.

Therapist: Say, "I must be strong so that..." Put an ending on it.

Client: I must be strong so that I don't start crying.

Therapist: Finish this: "If I ever started crying..." or "If I ever expressed my sadness..."

Therapist: Repeat after me, "I feel it is all right for me to feel/act sexual." Is that statement true or false? Let's discuss it now.

Client: I don't feel as vulnerable as before.

Therapist: That's how you *don't* feel. Tell me how you do feel now.

Therapist: "If I ever let anyone know my true feelings..." Put an ending on it. Begin.

Client: If I ever...

Therapist: Again. A different ending on it.

(REPEAT SEVERAL TIMES.)

Client: (looking sad, ready to cry)

Therapist: Close your eyes. Can you stay with that feeling? Your eyes are welling up with tears.

(This is a good time to induce hypnosis, when the subconscious is open and receptive—when feelings are being expressed.)

Body Awareness

Client: I'm scared.

Therapist: Go into your body. Where do you feel scared?

Client: In my hands.

Therapist: Go into your hands. How do your hands feel? Say, "They feel as though..." "They feel as if..."

Client: I feel confused.

Therapist: Separate the confusion. Say, "On one hand I feel _____ and on the other hand I feel _____."

(This can then be turned into Gestalt dialogue, with one part talking to another part.)

Client: I feel stuck.

Therapist: That's an impasse. Say, "On one hand..."

Client: It overcomes me. (Or, It isn't working.)

Therapist: There is no "it." Say, "I."

Client: I feel helpless.

Sentence Completions

Therapist: Close your eyes. I'm going to point out possible benefits to maintaining the status quo. I would like you to think about each one, and we'll discuss it. Repeat after me and finish the sentence.

1. I attract sympathy and attention by...

2. I can control and dominate the behavior of others by...

3. I punish myself for real and imagined sins by...

4. I punish someone else by...

5. I avoid the responsibility of...

REEDUCATION AND REPROGRAMMING

Reproducing the Initial Sensitizing Event

Client believed he suffered from "tardive dyskinesia"—in hypnotic age regression his tongue stuck to the roof of his mouth. He thought he was suffocating to death because of his panic.

Therapist: One, two, three. Now your mouth is drying, drying up, and you feel as if you're choking. Tell me your name. (Client can't speak.)

Changing the Memory

Let your mind grow clear and your mouth grow moist. This time I am going to send you back there and you will be calm and in control even when I tell you your mouth is growing dry. The dryness will be a temporary situation you can overcome.

Decontaminating a Feeling Memory

Fear of roller coaster rides.

Client is in trance.

Therapist: Go back to the time you went on the ride. Now experience the crowds, the screaming, the physical sensations you had. Now let your mind grow clear.

Therapist: Now, go back in time to the top of the roller coaster, before the descent, knowing that this time you will be calmer. The thought will be in your mind, "It will soon be over. I can live through this." Now the roller coaster is starting, the crowd is shouting and screaming, and you are thinking, "I am calmer, I can live through this." Now let your mind grow clear.

Now, go back to the top of the ride again. This time when you take the ride, you will be bathed by a white light during the ride. Your creative intelligence will keep you calm and comfortable. The ride is beginning, and the white light surrounds and protects you. You are remaining calm and comfortable.

Go into yourself and give a report.

Reprogramming

Example 1:

Therapist: Whenever you feel your old negative feelings returning, cross your fingers, breathe deeply, and say:

"Calm, poised, and free."

Now, let the relaxation come upon you so you can function easily with confidence. These suggestions are more powerful than your old ways of thinking because you realize they are based on truth.

(REPEAT SEVERAL TIMES.)

Example 2:

Therapist: Imagine a control panel in your brain. There are many switches, dials, and knobs. The knobs on the control panel have numbers from one to ten. One knob, marked "Pain," increases or decreases your pain as it is turned clockwise or counterclockwise. Ten is intense pain and zero is total freedom. Now start turning the knob marked "Pain" down to zero, and feel the pain growing less as you click the knob into lower numbers.

Now go into your body and give a report.

Healing Suggestions

Therapist: The creative intelligence within you made a perfect body for you that knows how to restore and rejuvenate you. It can heal you when you get a cut and stop healing when the healing of the cut is complete. This is as God and nature intended it to be. The healing power is within you and you know that. Unlike other animals, you have the ability to interfere with the divine plan, with the natural healing that occurs. You do this by reacting to a traumatic event in such a way that it reprograms your subconscious to cause symptoms that continue to affect you today, even though there is no need for these symptoms in your daily life.

Bioenergetics Techniques Used in Trance

Use your arm as "neck." Place client's hands on arm and give instructions to squeeze, to choke your forearm. Instruct the client to shout:

Client: I hate you!

I'll kill you!

(ALTERNATE REPEATEDLY.)

Therapist: Go into your body. Give a report.

Infantile Protest Through Alternate Kicking

Therapist: You are lying on your back. Each time I speak to you, raise your legs alternately and kick down into the couch and say "No!" or "No, I won't!" Now start kicking.

Client: No.

Therapist: Yes.

Client: No I won't.

Therapist: Yes you will. Do as I say.

Client: No! I won't!

Therapist: Listen to your mother.

Client: No I won't!

Therapist: Go to your room, now.

Client: No I won't!

Therapist: Shut up.

Client: No, I won't!

Therapist: Do as you're told.

Client: No, I won't!

Therapist: Now rest. Tend to your breathing. Go into your body. Give a report. Start kicking again.

Client: You scare me! (ALTERNATE WITH:)

Client: I resent you!

(ALTERNATE REPEATEDLY.)

Therapist: Now rest. Go into your body. Give a report. Start kicking again.

Shout "I hate you!"

Shout "I'll kill you!" (ALTERNATE REPEATEDLY.)

Now rest. Go into your body. Give a report.

GESTALT DIALOGUES

Dialogue With Significant Others at Time of Sensitizing Event

Therapist: This time when I count to three, your father (mother, etc.) is seated in a chair about six feet in front of you, and you are seated in a chair facing him (her, etc.).

One, two, three. There sits your (father). I want you to talk to (him) now. How would you address (him)? Do you call (him) (Dad, Daddy, Father)?

Say, "(Dad), I want to talk to you. I want to tell you my true feelings." Now tell (him.) (Wait for statement of feeling to begin. Then say:)

Now I want you to change places. Be the (father). Answer your (son/daughter). Speak to your (son/daughter) who says (he/she) feels this way about you.

Be the (son/daughter). Answer your (father).

Body Part Dialogue

Therapist: Let your mind grow clear.

Separate yourself into two parts. Be the (head) and be the (chest). Be the pain in your (chest). Talk to your (head). Say: "I am the pain in the (chest)."

Inanimate Object Dialogue

Client: I say yes to everything. I'm just a doormat.

Therapist: Be a doormat. Give your size, shape, color, purpose, function. Start with, "I am a doormat and..."

Emotions

Client: I feel fearful.

Therapist: Describe the fear. Now be the fear and describe yourself.

Fear: I keep you stuck, vulnerable.

Therapist: Tell (client's name) "You need me" and why.

Fear: You need me to hold you back.

Therapist: Be (client's name)'s heart. Talk to the fear.

Death Fantasy

Client: I wish I were dead.

Therapist: Imagine you are dead. You are in the coffin before burial. Your (mother) is looking down on you. What is (she) saying, thinking, or feeling?

Revoking Childhood Promises

Therapist: Hold out your arms. Say, "(Mama), where are you? I need you. Why don't you love me? I'm a good (girl)." Tell (her) what it will be like when you grow up: "(Mama), when I grow up..." Put an ending on it.

Start again...another ending. Another... Another... Now start kicking again and reverse those promises.

Example:

Client: Mama, when I grow up, I won't be like you.

Power Programming

Therapist: There are many people who want to love you but you don't accept their love. You *feel* alone and abandoned but the truth is that you are loved and you are lovable!

Repeat after me! I eagerly accept the love that surrounds me now, and I am filled and nourished by it.

Woman's Sexual Affirmation

Therapist: Repeat after me!

I have a right to sexual happiness.

I have a divine right to happiness.

I accept myself as a lovable person.

I easily accept love and approval.

I easily express my love to others.

I love my body.

I love the pleasure I find in my body.

I am a loving woman.

I have a right to sexual happiness.

Daughter's Affirmation to Psychosexual Needs of Father

(For sexual sensitizing, victims of incest or sexual abuse, sexually jealous parent, etc. Also used in Gestalt dialogue with abuser.)

Therapist: Repeat after me!

I have the right to love other men.

I have the right to accept love from other men.

It is not my responsibility to make you sexually happy.

It is not my obligation to be the object of your sexual desire.

I want you to live, but I cannot be responsible for your life.

Only you are responsible for your living.

Living Up to Someone's Expectations

Speak to father/mother/husband, etc.

I'll no longer let you ruin my life.

Therapist: Repeat after me:

I no longer need to live up to your expectations, and you no longer need to live up to my expectations of you.

I give up these expectations of you because I know it is unlikely you will change.

You can go on doing what you've always done, but my attitude will be different.

If we can ever discover each other as unique human beings it would be wonderful.

But if that never happens, I can accept that too, for that's the way it is.

Reaffirming Positive Feelings and Values

Therapist: I am going to give you some words to focus on. They are:

Peace and contentment

Go to a time and place that has to do with these feelings of peace and contentment. To help you get there more quickly, squeeze your right hand into a fist. When you experience these feelings, raise your right arm and squeeze your fist tighter. Now let your arm fall back into your lap, and let these feelings fall back into your memory.

Beauty

Go to a time and place that has to do with beauty... Let beautiful thoughts and feelings fill you now!

Joy

Go to a time and place that has to do with a joyful time and feeling... Let feelings of joy fill you now.

Love

(An antidote to self-hatred.)

Go to a time and place when you feel loved and lovable, when you feel loving... Let loving feelings fill you now! (Pause for thirty seconds. Begin again.)

If you aren't experiencing peace and contentment, it does not mean these feelings do not exist. You simply are not allowing them to flow through you. When you feel ugliness around you, it does not mean that there is no beauty. We are surrounded by beauty all the time. You are not allowing yourself to experience beauty. When you are enveloped in sadness, it does not mean there is no joy in life. You are not allowing yourself to experience the joy of living. When you do not feel love, it does not mean there is no love available to you. You simply are not open to it.

These are divine qualities given to you to glorify the Creative Source. From this time forward, you are developing a powerful belief in your ability to use your divine faculties and to express these human qualities. You accept yourself as a lovable person because you are lovable. Repeat after me:

I accept myself as a lovable person.

I easily express love, affection, and approval.

I eagerly and joyously accept the love, affection, and approval that surround me now.

I am filled and nourished by the love and approval that surround me.

I deserve love for I am loving and I am lovable.

I am unique.

I have special qualifications.

I am important to life.

Never before has life been expressed through any other person in exactly the same way it is expressed by me.

For if it were, there would be no need for me to be here.

I have a special place in the scheme of life.

I approve of myself as a loving person.

Now go inside yourself and see what you are feeling and what you experience. When you are ready, give a report.

PRE-TRANCE TERMINATION

Therapist: In a moment I'm going to bring you back into full conscious awareness. Before I do, is there anything further you want to say to me or ask me or tell me today?

Rationale: To ensure that the client does not feel "unfinished."

Therapist: Quickly now, who do I remind you of?

Rationale: To determine psychic identification (transference).

Therapist: What qualities do I share with _____?

Rationale: To separate qualities versus persona.

POST-TRANCE TERMINATION

Review the trance through client's feedback

Therapist: You really surprised yourself, didn't you? Tell me about it.

(Wait for client's report.)

Set the climate for the next session with post-hypnotic suggestion

Therapist: You will sleep well tonight and be ready for the next session.

You will gain many insights during this coming week.

(When an impasse develops and the client seems "stuck," you can bring the client out of hypnosis, saying:)

Therapist: This week you will have many uncomfortable feelings, but you can cope with them. You'll feel your conflict attempting to resolve itself. Let your creative intelligence help you to go past being "stuck."

You are going to dream and solve these problems. Your creative intelligence will help you.

You are going to sleep poorly with lots of dreaming. Your subconscious mind will use this time to bring you through the impasse.

Give an assignment for the next session

Therapist: You are to give at least three compliments each day... (Describe and explain assignment.)

Address the will to fail: Trying is lying

When you give an assignment and the client seems hesitant, or says "I'll try," explain that trying implies failure. It is a built-in excuse. "Well, I tried." Explain the concept of time:

Therapist: We can only use time. We cannot make it, waste it, or kill it. Each person has twenty-four hours in the day, no more and no less. There's no such thing as not having enough time. It is up to us to use our time effectively and to set priorities!

If there is continued resistance, use threat of termination:

Therapist: If I give you 100 percent of myself as your therapist and you are unwilling to give 100 percent of yourself, it's time to end our sessions until you are ready for a greater commitment to change. Shall we talk about it now?

Factors that Create Readiness for Change

Readiness for change depends on:

1. the creative value of suffering—mental, physical, or emotional/psychic. (When we have suffered enough we can overcome our fear of change.)

2. overwhelming anxiety triggering either life-affirming (reaching out for help) or life-negating (entering into addictions) activity.

3. the realization that change is possible by mobilizing and using one's own inner power. (Our altered perception enables us to overcome a conditioned disbelief in our ability to use our inner power creatively.)

Primary movements of the Subconscious Mind

1. *The movement away from pain*, which is linked to our survival mechanism. We develop a conditioned tolerance to physical and emotional pain (masochism). We become accustomed to pain and it becomes our normal existence.

2. *The movement toward pleasure.* The movement away from pain is always stronger than the movement toward pleasure (the basis for all addictions).

The knowledge of a *diagnosis*, or naming a *symptom* allows a client to avoid responsibility. As long as the symptom persists, he doesn't have to function. Clients will accept a medical diagnosis sooner than a psychiatric diagnosis.

When an emotionally induced symptom persists for an extended length of time, it can produce an organic change.

Feed back the words the client needs to hear. When he feels powerless, point out his strengths and inner power when he is in trance. Be indirect in the beginning, and gradually increase your focus on the client's strength.

No matter how much the client reveals, most of the psyche will remain a mystery. Never assume you have all the answers.

Deal with what emerges!

This is the most important rule in hypnotherapy. Don't try to psychoanalyze! Don't be a "rescuer" (savior); don't try to force change! Work creatively and allow change to happen. Listen to the voice quality. Watch the body language carefully.

Body Armoring (Wilhelm Reich)

Clients may use a part of the body as an armor against feeling, for example, jutting out the chin as a physical attempt to keep from crying, or a lump in the throat which restricts breathing. Restricted breathing lessens the oxygen supply needed for heightened feeling, and thus prevents the emergence of intense feeling.

An example of complementary unconscious needs is when a woman's maternalism and succorance is complemented by her husband's need for a mother figure. When a child is born, the husband is displaced and feels neglected and resentful.

To get rid of introjected feelings, clients may vomit or have diarrhea. Dry heaves happen during therapy as clients rid themselves of introjected feelings:

"He makes me sick."

"I just can't stomach it."

"She turns my stomach when _____."

"It really gripes me when _____."

If clients begin to cry intensely, let them cry for as long as they need to. Say "Stay with the feeling." Do not give tissues for "mopping up" or try to close down their crying until the session is over.

In age regression, clients are not reliving an experience, they are remembering it with great emotional intensity and vivid clarity.

Help clients to understand a relationship; do not criticize it. Everyone is *innocent even when they are guilty*. If father had sexual feelings towards his daughter, it may be that he felt unlovable and sought the uncritical acceptance of the child. *Do not poison the relationship* with Dad by saying he was sick, wrong, or evil—especially if he is still alive. Actual reconciliation may not be possible, but the client must learn to reconcile her psychic rage, fear, and ambivalent feelings for her own personal development.

OTHER USEFUL IDEAS AND CONCEPTS

The Process

When testing in hypnosis, always use the *subjunctive mood*. In arm levitation, say, "*It feels as though* your arm is just too heavy too lift." This thought is acceptable to both the conscious and unconscious mind. "You cannot lift your arm!" is often heard as a challenge to the ego.

The goal is not to get the client into a trance. The goal is to do the best possible work in a therapy session. *The trance symbolizes the acceptance of the contract of trust.* Continue to establish trust through a nonjudgmental, accepting attitude of unconditional love. When the client shows the need to defy, to reject, to seduce, show no negative response. Continue your positive acceptance: "That's fine. Now we're going to...."

It is the therapist's role to penetrate and dissipate the client's resistance. You steal the client's time and money when you tell him he is a difficult subject. It is the therapist who has a problem, not the client.

Client resistance is a test. When you fail the test, creative therapy ends, in principle if not in actuality. Many clients expect you to fail the test, especially if they have been in therapy before without creative results.

Do not give *hypnotic programming suggestions* until the client is ready. When induction is difficult, trust is not yet established. The client will not accept and follow any suggestions unless he trusts the wisdom of his therapist.

Hypnotized clients produce a mixture of reality, fantasy, and dreams. Much of this is recorded in the mind as historical events. But the memory is the reality of psychic existence. It doesn't matter if the events are truly historical. The psychic effect is the same.

Carl Rogers notes that the therapist must *learn to be gullible*. Accept what your client says. You are not in the lie detection business. When the client presents a paradox, point it out to him for clarification, saying, "Three weeks ago you said _____. Now you are saying _____. It seems there's a paradox. Let's discuss it."

When you start from a very permissive position, it is difficult to switch to an authoritarian role. Start from strength, from authority. You can always soften if you come up against someone who fears authoritarian relationships.

Therapist: *HYPNOSIS* creates mental and physical relaxation which allows your subconscious mind to accept and respond to creative and beneficial ideas.

Therapist: I will act as a guide to help you be good to yourself so that you won't need to sabotage yourself anymore.

Therapist: You could resist if you chose to; that's not why you're here.

The Critical Factor

When someone tells you what you *should* do, he is usually working through his own feelings, through his Critical Parent, rather than responding as an adult.

The critical factor is fully developed by age eleven. Until then, the child interprets each message literally, viz., "You'll be the death of me." We live out that role, script, or attribution throughout our lifetime as a self-fulfilling prophecy.

Prior to the development of the critical factor, the subconscious has no sense of humor. Everything is taken literally. By age fifty, the man who had been told repeatedly by his father that he "had no guts" had already had half of his intestines removed surgically.

When we experience a trauma, or *sensitizing event*, the critical factor is temporarily blown aside and the non-analytic subconscious mind creates an emotionalized belief that can dominate our adult life.

When a parent says, "If you hadn't been so naughty, that wouldn't have happened to you," the subconscious mind translates it as *"God fixed you."*

When you say, "I'm not going to be like my (mother/father)," you create and focus on what you don't want. The subconscious mind uses every means at its disposal to bring the mental blueprint into your life.

Implementing Change

We can only experience change by initiating a process of change, not by talking or thinking about it. If that's all it took, the hungry could be fed by thoughts of food.

Because we hate that which we fear, we invest it with great energy. This is the basis for Job's great psychological discovery, "The thing that I have greatly feared has come upon me."

When you grow up without a positive model in your life, you focus only on what you don't want to be, instead of what you want to be.

Only human beings have a continuing capacity for change. All other animals can act only out of programmed instinct. We don't expect a pig to catch a mouse in the barn.

"Be transformed by the renewing of your mind."
"Be ye transformed in a twinkling of an eye." —*St. Paul*

The Intellectual Mind vs. the Feeling Mind

Intellectual awareness does not trigger a therapeutic response. Knowledge of what we do and why we do it does not free us to change our lives. The intellect alone is always ineffective in stimulating transformation.

We need to develop organismic awareness—not the "why" of what we are doing, but the "what" and "how." "Post facto" awareness means discovering that we repeat the same behavior again and again and always regret it after the fact. We need awareness *before* we repeat the mistake. Knowing "why" does not keep anyone from repeating the mistake. We can always block conscious awareness so that we can repeat mistakes and rationalize them.

We spend our lives doing what we feel like doing. When the feeling mind and the intellectual mind are in conflict, the feeling mind wins out. Hypnotherapy brings our feeling mind into alignment with our intellectual mind. The *mystical marriage* is the linking together of the intellect and the feeling mind. Sometimes the intellect may overrule the feelings to avoid painful consequences, such as keeping us from telling the boss off when he makes us angry. In the case of obesity and alcoholism, the intellect knows this life-negating behavior is wrong, but the feelings win, and we continue to eat or drink because it makes us feel good or temporarily stops us from feeling bad. When the intellect takes over to implode feelings, the imaginative function can become intensely negative, leading to feelings of hopelessness. Hopelessness leads to despair, which then leads to anti-life behavior in the form of either fast suicide or slow suicide through alcoholism, drug addiction, obesity, or compulsive sexuality.

Compulsive overeating, drug taking, and similar behaviors are an effort to insulate us from the "slings and arrows of outrageous fortune."

The imagination is our source of hope. We can imagine the coming together of elements in our life that will bring happiness by helping us to fill our deepest needs.

On Feelings and Emotions

When we dread the love relationship, we select someone for whom there is little possibility of developing strong feelings of attachment so that we can cut that person off without feeling a sense of loss. In that way, we can reject the love object first. When we seek out someone we can really love, it is always far more painful to be rejected by them.

Our feelings of unlovability are a form of self-hatred. Who else would we treat as meanly as we treat ourselves?

Too good to be true means you don't think you deserve better, or that you don't deserve to be helped.

The paradox is that we are always surrounded by love. It takes a great deal of energy to continue to feel unlovable when we are surrounded by love. We don't create new energy to transform ourselves. We need only to liberate the energy we have invested in our painful existence, so that we can redirect it into life-affirming behavior.

We learn to love by being loved and accepting that love. Knowing we are loved is the most important lesson learned in childhood.

This is the essence of the *neurotic love pact:* "I will pretend you are the only woman in the world if you pretend I am the only man, and we will fulfill all of each other's needs." An impossible task!

Obsessive jealousy is made up of a natural desire to be loved and be lovable, and an unnatural belief that we are not loved and are unlovable!

"I hate people" can be translated "I reject them before they reject me, then they won't have the opportunity to discover that I am unlovable."

The Unspeakable Truth: "I am unlovable."

There is only one phobia—fear of being unlovable.

People pleasers are exploited for their weakness, for their need to feel love and approval. You can stop people-pleasing by being assertive, by asking for what you want. However, *assertion* is not limited to one certain emotion. You can assert yourself quietly and gently, forcefully and loudly, or with anger and hostility. Assertion speaks to the issue of what you want and need, what you will accept, and what you won't accept.

You never learn to say YES until you learn to say the word NO. Otherwise, Yes is usually a disguised No. Once you want to say No and can say No, the Yeses that follow come from the heart.

Shyness appears socially acceptable but it really is not. Adult shyness is a fear-based determination surrounded by a great sea of anger. "If you want to make contact with me, you'll take the first step because I never do." It's a control mechanism. Shy people are concerned they are not attracting the kind of people they want, which inflames their powerful feelings of resentment.

On expressing feelings... There's a difference between feeling you want to hit someone and actually hitting them—thought versus action. You can say, "You make me so angry I feel like hitting you." This can lead into constructive, rather than destructive, dialogue.

Withholding is a form of deceit. If I don't let you know how I'm feeling, I'm deceiving you.

You don't always need to act on your feelings—simply acknowledge them and set yourself free. Be honest and show your feelings when you feel them. There can be consequences to "letting it all hang out." Be sure the time, place and situation are appropriate when you "tell it like it is." The price may be more than you expected to pay.

There are four classes of primary feelings:
    anger—resentment, rage
    sadness—self-pity
    joy—euphoria
    sexual feelings—orgasm

Feelings can be exploded or imploded. Allowing some feelings to explode keeps us in touch with reality. Imploded feelings lead to depression, withdrawal, and eventually to catatonia. People who withhold feelings often use sexual expression as the only means to "explode."

For example, Marilyn Monroe is quoted as saying, "I only feel alive when I'm balling." Her other feelings were powerfully imploded and unavailable to her. Her sexual intensity was her measurement of her participation in life.

We can't fill all of our own needs. We do need others. *Sadness* is normal when we experience a loss of someone who helped fill our needs.

We are the only ones who can mark our own scorecards because we set our own standards. We can approve of ourselves rather than seek approval from others who get their information secondhand from us.

If you appreciate yourself as a mature adult, you don't need to continue waiting for Mommy or Daddy to appreciate you. You can nurture yourself. What are you going to do to be good to yourself, and when will you start?

The Power of the Divine

My spiritual beliefs bring me reassurance, consolation, inspiration. Your atheism gives you nothing.

When you don't believe in God, you'll believe in anything.

When you don't believe in God enough, it's because you believe in your problems more.

"As a child, I thought as a child; I saw through a glass darkly. As a man, I see clearly; I put aside childish things." *1 Cor 13. St. Paul to the Corinthians*

THE "EXPERTS" ATTEMPT TO DEFINE *HYPNOSIS*

The greatest discovery of my generation is that human beings can alter their lives by altering their attitudes of mind.

William James

Actually, the hypnotic state, like the conscious state and the sleeping state, is extremely complex and involves so many physiological, psychological, and interpersonal factors that no one theory has yet been able to account for all the intricate operations that take place within its range.

Lewis R. Wolberg

Hypnosis is the term applied to a unique, complex form of unusual but normal behavior which can be induced in all normal persons under suitable conditions and also in many persons suffering from various types of abnormality. It is primarily a special psychological state with certain physiological attributes, resembling sleep only superficially and marked by a functioning of the individual at a level of awareness other than the ordinary conscious state...

Encyclopedia Britannica

Hypnotism is simply exaggerated suggestibility.

George H. Estabrooks

...A state of intensified attention and receptiveness, and an increased responsiveness to an idea or to a set of ideas.

Milton H. Erickson

...Nothing but an aspect of conditioning.

Andrew Salter

Hypnosis is largely a question of your willingness to be receptive and responsive to ideas, and to allow these ideas to act upon you without interference. These ideas we call suggestions.

Andre M. Weitzenhoffer
and Ernest R. Hilgard

Hypnosis is not sleep. Whatever sleep is, hypnosis is not....to put it succinctly, hypnosis is an altered state of attention which approaches peak concentration capacity.

Herbert Spiegel

Hypnosis is a consent state of physiological relaxation where the subject allows the critical censor of the mind to be bypassed to a greater, or lesser, degree...we could even go so far as to say that hypnosis is "preventive psychological medicine."

Peter Blythe

It is recognized that there is no generally accepted definition of hypnosis, though considerable consensus exists at a descriptive level.

Martin T. Orne

...An altered state within which suggestions have a peculiarly potent effect.

K. S. Bowers

Hypnosis is a natural state of mind with special identifying characteristics:

1. An extraordinary quality of relaxation.

2. An emotionalized desire to satisfy the suggested behavior: The person feels like doing what the hypnotist suggests, provided that what is suggested does not generate conflict with his belief system.

3. The organism becomes self-regulating and produces normalization of the central nervous system.

4. Heightened and selective sensitivity to stimuli perceived by the five senses and four basic perceptions.

5. Immediate softening of psychic defenses.

Gil Boyne

EXPERTS ADDRESS THE SAFETY OF HYPNOSIS

Leslie Le Crone, psychologist and authority on hypnotism, states, "As to self-induction, many thousands have learned it; and I have yet to hear a report of any bad results of its use."

In his book *Clinical and Experimental Hypnosis*, Dr. William S. Kroger states: "Platonof, an associate of Pavlov, who used hypnosis over fifty years in over fifty-thousand cases, reports as follows: 'We have never observed any harmful influences on the patient which could be ascribed to the method of hypno-suggestion therapy, or any tendency toward the development of unstable personality, weakening of the will, or pathological urge for hypnosis.'"

Dr. David Cheek, M.D., who has vast experience in the field, writes, "We can do more harm with ignorance of hypnotism than we can ever do by intelligently using hypnosis and suggestion constructively."

Dr. Julius Grinker states, "The so-called dangers from hypnosis are imaginary. Although I have hypnotized many hundreds of patients, I have never seen any ill effects from its use."

Pierre Janet, a student of Sigmund Freud who became an ardent practitioner of hypnosis, writes, "The only danger in hypnotism is that it is not dangerous enough."

Psychologist Rafael Rhodes, in his book *Therapy Through Hypnosis*, writes: "Hypnotism is absolutely safe. There is no known case on record of harmful results from its therapeutic use."

Dr. Louie P. Thorpe, Professor Emeritus, University of Southern California,.in his book *The Psychology of Mental Health*, writes: "Hypnotism is a natural phenomenon, and there are no known deleterious effects from its use."

David Spiegel, M.D., Professor of Psychiatry and Behavioral Sciences, Stanford University School of Medicine, put it this way: "Physicians often worry that hypnosis involves significant risks to patients. Actually, the phenomenon is not dangerous and has fewer side effects than even the most benign medications.

Clinical hypnotherapist Gil Boyne states, "In almost forty years of practice and more than 40,000 hours of hypnotherapy, I have never seen or heard of any harm resulting from hypnosis."

There has never been a single documented case of harm resulting from the use of hypnosis.

INDEX

Adult life: contaminated by early childhood programming 15

Adult Reasoning Mind: 50-51; 119-121; 288; 322; 325

Age Regression
19; 68,137; 210-215; 225-226; 275-290; 318-322
adult reasoning mind; 50-51; 119-122; 288; 322; 325
analyzing of, 50
childhood fears, 113
examining past behavior, 214-216
freedom from attribution, 35
Gestalt Dialogue, 72-86; 118-119; 226-234; 361-366; 319-322; 326-329; 336-339; 361-366
going further back: 115
indirect reeducation, 24; 26; 29
initial sensitizing event, 20; 24; 30; 45, 116; 152-153; 225; 250; 276 353
intensifying feeling, 21-22; 24, 30; 44; 45; 49; 67; 116; 152-153; 225; 250; 352; 275; 276; 353
looking back in dissociated manner, 146
reeducation, 22-23; 31-32; 50-54; 62-63; 146-150; 218-223; 234-241; 252-264; 290-301; 334
reprogramming, 31-32; 357-359
request for change, 34
: retroflection, 32
rewriting the imprint, 23
sensitizing event, 20; 24, 30; 45; 116; 152-153; 225; 250; 276; 353
subconscious selection, 218

Alcoholism: 198-case study, 187; 217

Altered perception: spelling problem, 36; 38

Ambivalent Feelings: 83

Anger Covers Hurt: 28

Assertion: expressed as defiance, 75

Attitude: paranoia, 192

Attitude: universe is malevolent, 192

Attribution:
fixed idea, 27
freedom from, 35
mental block, 23
weakening during trance, 28

Authority Figure: 128

Autonomy: need for, 74

Avoidance of responsibility: 40

Awareness: levels of, 313-314

Behavior pattern: recognizes avoidance, 33

Belief Development: 304-305

Bioenergetics: 359

Boyne, Gil: 3
age regression, 19; 68,137; 210-215; 225-226; 275-290; 318-322
assessing progress of client, 38-43; 58-62
assisting client identify feelings, 110-112; 116-117; 127
characteristics of, xi
classification of Instructional Programs Review Meeting, 5
client familiarity with hypnosis, 159-162
definition of hypnosis, 380-381
direct suggestion, 294-298
educating, 345-346
eliciting information from client, 16-18; 41-43; 59-62; 98-103; 110-112; 126-136; 156-162; 188-205; 244-264; 304-317
evaluating results: 35-37; 38-40; 55-57; 58-59; 90-92; 107-108; 152-153; 185; 215-216; 217-220; ,240-241; 272-274; 300-301; 344-346
extemporaneous speaking, 100
extemporaneous teaching, 100
Gestalt Dialogue, 48-50; 72-86; 118-119; 226-234; 319-322; 326-329; 336-339; 361-366

grounding client to feelings, 131-136

indirect re-education: 24-26; 29; 31

induction, 18-19; 43-44; 67; 103-104; 112-113; 136; 165-172; 205-206; 223-224; 264-269; 274; 317-318

infantile kicking, 83-84; 116; 140; 147-148; 151; 197; 316-317; 356-357

initial sensitizing event, 20; 24, 30; 45; 116; 132; 152-153; 225; 250; 276; 353

: initiating client's sentence, 83-84; 116; 140; 147-148; 151; 197, 316-317; 356-357

integration during trance, 35

intensifying feeling during trance, 20; 21-22; 24; 30; 45; 49; 67; 116; 152-153; 225; 250; 352; 275; 276; 353

on being stuck, 230

on programming children, 41

on resistance to change, 39

on returning to old pattern, 38

parts, use of, 276-278

practitioner and teacher, xiii

programming during trance, 35

reality in age regression: 55-57

reeducating, 22-23; 146-150; 218-223; 234-241; 252-264; 290-301; 334

safety of hypnosis, 383

secondary reinforcing event, 26

short term hypnotherapy, xi

spelling in trance state, 112-113; 136-137, 179; 209; 274-275

stuttering case study, 303

summarizes direct suggestion, 107-108

teaching, 315-316, 324, 340-341

weakening the attribution during trance, 28

"Busy": 131-132

Case Study:
  Alcoholism, 187
  Alcoholism, session one, 187
  Alcoholism, session two, 217
  Anger, 125
  Change of Lifestyle, 125
  Childhood Fears, 109
  Fear of Public Speaking, 97
  Finding Lost Objects, 155
  Impotence, 243
  Impotence, session two, 272
  Spelling, 15
  Stuttering, 303
  Stuttering, follow-up, 347

Change:
  implementing, 374
  process of 63
  readiness for, 369
  resistance to, 39
  William James, 39

Childhood fears: projection of, 109

Chiropractor: speech therapy, 309-310

Client's: assisting client identify feelings, 110-112

Compensation: 223

Conditional love: 74

Confidence: 188-189

Conscious effort: 258

Critical Factor: 373-374

Criticism: fear of, 24, 191

Cycle: mental block, 29

Definitions of Hypnosis: 379-381

Direct Gaze: Induction Technique, 112

Direct Suggestion: 294-298

Divine: power of, 378

Dream: 314

Eliciting Information from client, 16-
18; 41-43; 59-62; 98-103; 110-
112; 126-136; 156-162; 188-205;
244-264; 304-317; 354-357
Emotionally Based Belief: 25
Emotions and Feelings: 375-378
Emotions: intesifying, 20; 21-22; 24;
30, 44; 45; 49; 67; 116; 152-153;
225; 250; 352; 275; 276; 353
Energy: transformed, 189
Erection: physiology, 293
Erickson: Dr. Milton, xi
Evaluating the session: 35-37; 38-40;
55-57; 58-59; 90-92; 107-108;
152-153; 185; 215-216; 217-220;
240-241; 272-274; 300-301; 344-
346
Experts:
Define Hypnosis, 379-381
Safety of Hypnosis, 382-383

Fear of public speaking: 98
Feeling Mind: 374-375
Feeling:
intensifying, 20; 21-22; 24; 30; 44;
45, 49, 67; 116; 152-153; 225;
250; 352; 275; 276; 353
what others think, 88-91
Feelings and Emotions: 375-378
ambivalent, 83; withholding, 377
Finding lost objects: 155
Freedom, feeling of: 69-72; 86-88
Freud, Sigmund: 8; objections to
hypnotherapy, xiii

Gestalt Dialogue: 48-50; 72-86; 118-
119; 226-234; 281; 319-322; 326-
329; 336-339; 361-366
Goal Setting: 351
Good-bye, saying: 345
Grounding client's feelings: 131-136;
329; 336-339; 361-366

Hypnosis:
: adult reasoning mind, 50-51, 119-
122; 288; 322; 325
: age regression; see Age Regression
: case study, alcoholism, session one,
187
: case study, alcoholism, session two,
21
: case study, anger, 125
: case study, change of lifestyle, 125
: case study, childhood fears, 109
: case study, fear of public speaking,
97
: case study, finding lost objects, 155
: case study, impotence, 243
: case study, impotence, session two,
272
: case study, spelling, 15
: case study, stuttering, 303
: case study, stuttering, follow-up,
347
: god of sleep, 268
: direct gaze, 112
: client familiarity with hypnosis,
159-162
: critical factor, 373-374
: defined by experts, 379-383
: eliciting information, 16-18; 41-
43; 59-62; 98-103; 110-112; 126-
136; 156-162; 188-205, 244-264,
304-317
: evaluation of session, 35-37; 38-40;
55-57; 58-59; 90-92; 107-108;
152-153; 185; 215-216; 217-220,
,240-241, 272-274; 300-301, 344-
346
: experience with, 204
: feeling mind, 374-375
: Gestalt dialogue, 48-50; 72-86;
118-119; 226-234; 281; 319-322;
326-329; 336-339, 361-366;
: inductions, 18-19, 43-44, 67, 103-
104, 112-113, 135, 165-172, 205-

206, 264-269, 274, 317-318
: Infantile kicking, 83-84; 116; 140;
147-148; 151; 197, 316-317; 356-
357
: intellectual mind, 374-375
: intensifying feeling, 20, 21-22, 24,
30, 45, 49, 116, 152-153, 225;
250,276 353
memory recall, 185
parts, 329
pre-induction interview, 351
pre-trance termination, 367
psychiatrist, 261
reality in age regression, 55-57
reeducation, 22-23; 146-150; 218-
223; 234-241; 252-264; 290-301;
334
returning to consciousness, 183
rewriting the imprint, 23
safety of, 382-383
sentence initiation, 83-84; 116;
140; 147-148; 151; 197, 316-317;
356-357
sleep of nervous system, 162
spelling in trance, 112-113; 136-
137; 179-180; 181; 209; 274-275
testing for trance, 262; 269-271
the process, 372-373
trance state difficulty with,16
Hypnotherapist: DOT definition, 3
Hypnotherapist: true ministry, 8;
realm of the Spirit: 8
Hypnotherapy:
adult reasoning mind, 50-51; 119-
122; 288; 322; 325
age regression, 19; 68; 137; 210-
215; 225-226; 275-290; 318-322;
see also Age Regression
alcoholism case study
brings freedom from attribution, 35
case study, impotence, 243
case study, session two, 272
direct suggestion, 294-298

for public speaking , 104-107
DOT definition is non-medical, 4
eliciting information, 16-18; 41-43;
59-62; 98-103; 110-112; 126-136;
156-162; 188-205; 244-264; 304-
317; 354-357
evaluating session, 35-37; 38-40;
55-57; 58-59; 90-92; 107-108;
152-153; 185; 215-216; 217-220;
240-241; 272-274; 300-301; 344-
346
examining past behavior, 214-216
finding lost objects, 155
follow-up, 351
freedom feeling, 69-72
Gestalt dialogue, 48-50; 72-86; 118-
119; 226-234; 319-322; 326
indirect reeducation: 26
inductions; see Inductions
hopeful work, xii
identify feelings, 116-117
indirect reeducation, 24, 26
infantile kicking, 83-84; 116; 140;
147-148; 151; 197; 316-317; 356-
357
initial sensitizing event, 20; 24; 30;
45; 116; 152-153; 225; 250; 276;
353
initiating a sentence for a client, 83-
84; 116; 140; 147-148; 151; 197;
316-317; 356-357
intensifying feeling: 20; 21-22; 24;
30; 45; 49; 67; 116; 152-153; 225;
250; 275; 276; 352; 275; 276; 352;
353
licensing,4
mental blocks, 15
non-licensed profession, 4
on being stuck, 230
parts therapy, 329-331
post-trance termination, 367-371
pre-trance termination, 367
public speaking, 98...

---

public speaking, 104-107
reeducation, 22-23; 26; 62-63; 146-
150; 234-241; 290-301; 334; 340-
341; 357-359
reprogramming, 357-361
request for change, 34
retroflection, 32
rewriting the imprint, 23
sensitizing event, 353
sentence initiating,83-84; 116; 135;
140; 147-148; 151; 197, 311; 316-
317; 356-357
short term therapy, xiii
spelling problem follow-up, 93-96
spelling, use of, 112-113; 136-13;
179; 209; 274-275
stuttering follow-up, 347
stuttering, 303
subconscious selection, 218
summarizing direct suggestion, 107-
108
Training Program Description: 5
training graduate schools of psychology, xiii
training medical schools, xiii
United States Government, 5
vs. Psychotherapy: 10-11
Hypnotic Session:
Spelling, No. 1, 16
Spelling, No. 2, 38...
Spelling, No. 3, 58
Gestalt Dialogue, 48-50; 72-86;
118-119; 319-322; 326-329; 336-
339; 361-366; 226-234
Hypnotism: boundless possibilities, ix-
x
natural power, ix
practical science, ix
practice of not prohibited, 4
Hypnotist: study of, ix

Identification: transference, 122, 151
Imagery: 314

Impotence:
Case study, 243
Session two, 272
Indirect Reeducation: 26, 31
Inductions, Hypnosis: 18-19; 27; 43-
44; 67; 103-104; 112-113; 136;
165-172; 205-206; 223-224; 264-
269; 274; 317-318
Infantile Kicking: 76; 359
Inferiority vs. goal settings: 223
Initial sensitizing event: 20; 22; 24;
30; 45; 116; 152-153; 225; 250;
317-318; 353
Insomnia: 219
Integration: 25; 35
spelling problem, 33
Intellectual Mind: 374-375
Intensifying the feeling: 20; 21-22; 24;
30; 45; 49; 67; 116; 152-153; 225;
250; 352; 275; 276; 353

James, William: on change, 39
Jealousy: 376
"Just Imagining": 310

Kappas, John: 3
Kicking, Infantile: 83-84; 116; 140;
147-148; 151; 197, 316-317; 356-
357
Knepflar, Dr. Kenneth: Speech pathologist, 309

Laughter: releases tension, 99
Lifestyle: change of, 125

Marx, Karl: 8
Medical schools: hypnotherapy
training, xiii
Memory recall: stimulating, 185
Mental Block:
and hypnotherapy, 15
attribution, 23, 27
fear of criticism, 24

cycle, 29
reinforcement, 25
rewriting the imprint, 23
self-fulfilling prophecy, 29
self-reinforcement, 27
spelling, 15
Mind: nature of, 268
Mistakes: as stepping stones, 233-234

Nature of Mind: 268
Negative belief: overcomes rules,28
Nervous system: response, 259
Neurohypnosis: 268

Other Useful Ideas and Concepts:
    372-378
    The process, 372-373
    The critical factor, 373-374
    Implementing change, 374
    The intellectual mind vs. the feeling
        mind, 374-375
    On feelings and emotions, 375-378
    The power of the divine, 378
Overcompensation: 223

Paranoia: 192
Parts Therapy: use of, 276-278; 329-
    331
Pattern:
    playing dumb, 196
    reasons for clinging to, 42-43
    secondary gains, 42
Paying the price: 43
Perfect: 336
Perfectionism: 62; 322
Performance anxiety: 101
Phenomena of trance: 10
Phobic avoidance: 79
Playing dumb: 196
Post-hypnotic suggestion: 367-368
Post-Trance Termination: 367-371
Power of Divine: 378
Pre-Induction Interview: 351

Pre-Trance Termination: 367
Predominant feeling: intensifying, 10;
    21-22; 24; 30; 44; 45; 49; 67; 116;
    152-153; 225; 250; 352; 275; 276;
    353
Pressure to learn: resistance: 17
Price to pay for not changing: 40
Primary Feelings: 377
Primary Movements: subconscious
    mind, 369-370
Professor on Hypnotherapy for stut-
    terers: 309
Programming: 35
Programming
    and Reeducation: 31-32
    children: 41
Prophecy: self-fulfilling, 259
Prostrate Gland: function, 263-264
Psychiatrist:
    hypnosis, 261
    speech therapy: 308
Psychoanalysis:
    pessimistic, xii
    scientific theory, 8
Psychoanalytic Assumptions: under-
    mining of traditional assump-
    tions, 7-9
Psychotherapy
    vs. Hypnotherapy: 10-11
    secular humanism, 8
Public Speaking:
    direct suggestion, 104-107
    fear of, 98
    vs. private speaking, 98

Rapport Building: 259
Readiness for Change: 369
Reality in age regression: 55-57
Reasoning Mind: retroflection, 32
Reeducation: 22-23; 62; 146-150;
    218-223; 234-241; 252-264; 290-
    301; 334; 340; 357-359

and Indirect Programming: 22-23;
42-43
weakening the attribution, 28
Regrets: a silliness, 219; 220
Reich, Wilhelm: 370
Reinforcing ridicule and embarrass-
ment: 27
Rejection: intense fear of, 190
Repression: 252
Reprogramming: 357-361
Resistance to change: 39; price to pay,
40
Response
pattern: development, 28
nervous system, 259
Responsibility, avoidance of: 40
Retroflection: 32
Rote learning vs. subconscious: 27

Safety of Hypnosis, 382-383
Scaring of self: 124
Secondary
gains: 42
payoff: 30
integration, 26
Self-criticism: 310
Self-esteem: 187
Self-fulfilling Prophecy: 29; 259
Sensitizing Event: 20; 24; 30; 45; 116;
152-153; 225; 250; 276; 353
Sentence Completions: 83-84; 116;
140; 147-148; 151; 197; 316-317;
356-357
Shyness: 377
Significant Statement, 20
age regression: 59; 69; 72
Similar Experience: rapport, 259
Speech Therapy:
chiropractor, 309-310
temporary results: 308
theories on, 307
Spelling problem, 16, 38, 58
a delusion 16

adult reinforcement, 30
follow-up, 93-96
freedom from attribution, 35
integration, 33
old pattern returning: 38
pattern of avoidance, 33
request for change, 34
secondary payoff, 33
self-reinforcement, 27
sensitizing event, 20
significant statement, 20
statement of altered perception, 36
two week progress report, 63, 64,
66-67
Spelling: use of in hypnosis, 112-113;
136-137; 179-181; 209; 274-275
Stammering vs. Stuttering: 305
Stimulating memory recall: 185
Stuttering vs. Stammering: 305
Stuttering:
case study, 303
everyone does so, 306
follow-up, 347
Subconscious fear: intensifying, 275
Subconscious feeling,: changing of, 73
Subconscious Mind:
blueprint, 293
feeling mind, 314
primary movements, 369-370
response: 258
Supreme Creator: 8

Techniques:
Pre-induction, 351
Goal setting, 351
Follow-up sessions, 351
Intensifying feelings, 352
Age regression, 353
Sensitizing event: 353
Information gathering, 354-356
Body awareness, 356
Sentence completions, 356-357

Reeducation and Programming, 357-361
Reproducing initial sensitizing event, 357
Changing the memory, 357
Decontaminating a feeling memory, 357-358
Reprogramming, 358-359
Healing suggestions, 359
Bioenergetics in trance, 359
Infantile protest, 360-361
Gestalt Dialogues, 361-366
With others at initial event, 361
Body part dialogue, 361
Inanimate object dialogue, 362
Emotions, 362
Death fantasy, 362
Revoking childhood promises, 362-363
Power programming, 363
Woman's sexual affirmation, 363
Daughter's affirmation to psychosexual needs of father, 364
Living up to someone's expectations, 364
Reaffirming positive feelings and values, 365-366
Pre-Trance Termination, 367
Post-Trance Termination, 367-371
Review the trance through the client's feedback, 367

Post-hypnotic suggestion, 367-368
Give assignment, 368
Trying is lying, 368
Factors that create readiness for change, 369
Primary movements of the secondary mind, 369-367
Deal with what emerges, 370
Body armoring, 370-371
Testing for Trance: 262
Traditional psychoanalytic assumption #1: 7; #2: 7; #3: 8-9
Trance feeling:
difficulty with, 16
intensifying, 19
Phenomena: 10
testing for, 269-271
Transference of identity, 151; 122
Transformation of energy: 189
Trying: lying, 193

Uncovering Techniques: 352
Unexpressed Rage: 326
Unreality, veil of, 31

Veil lifted: 31

Withholding Feelings: 377
Whetmore, California Senator James, 4

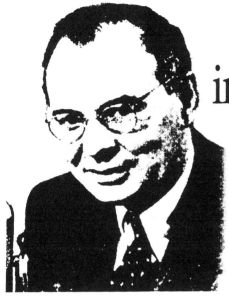

WESTWOOD PUBLISHING CO.
Books and audio/video products

THE HANDBOOK OF BRIEF PSYCHOTHERAPY BY HYPNOANALYSIS
By John A. Scott, Sr., Ph.D. - Soft Cover-280pp - $19.97
This book presents information beyond hypnosis into the theory and practice of advanced hypnotherapy. Why people have emotional problems and the causes and procedures of treatment. How hypnoanalysis enables people to change and the theoretical and philosophical concepts that underlie the process.

SELF HYPNOSIS & OTHER MIND EXPANDING TECHNIQUES
By Charles Tebbetts Soft Cover.139pp - $12.95
A practical and comprehensive guide to the use of self-hypnosis, autosuggestion, and subconscious reprogramming for self- improvement. This new, enlarged edition includes special sections on Weight Control and Stopping Smoking. A best seller.

HYPNOTHERAPY   By Dave Elman - Hard Cover.336pp - $39.95
Hailed as a classic in its field. Elman's major work is a forceful and dynamic presentation of hypnosis as a lightning-fast and amazingly effective tool in a wide range of therapies. A useful and practical summation of the teachings of one of the pioneers in hypnotherapy. Elman trained more physicians to use hypnosis than anyone before or since.

HYPNOSIS: The Mind/Body Connection   By Peter Mutke M.D. - Soft Cover-192pp - $14.95
A step-by-step series of easily understood procedures for making contact with and between our various physical and mental parts and functions so we may gain more control over our own health. Includes pain control, accelerated healing, weight reduction and more.

HYPNO-ANALYSIS   By Dave Elman - 6 audio cassettes + 68pp manual - $99.50
These extraordinary session in hypno-analysis consist of recordings of actual live therapy sessions presented by Dave Elman to physicians and psychiatrists. It is a rare opportunity to learn from the man who taught hypnotherapy to more healing arts professionals than any other instructor. Consists of six sessions of hypno-analysis explained and analyzed by Dave Elman.

PROFESSIONAL STAGE HYPNOTISM By Ormond McGill - Soft Cover 203pp - $14.95
A one-of-a-kind classic work, which covers all aspects of hypnotism demonstration. Includes a thorough look at all aspects of entertaining with hypnotism, including showmanship, presentations, staging, securing subjects, and dozens of thrilling routines. A wonderful vista of entertainment that can be performed for all occasions. This book prepares you with specific directions, instructions and routines whether demo in the living room for friends or on stage in a nightclub or theater.

HYPNO- VISION By Lisette Scholl - Soft Cover 197pp - $14.95
The Hypno- Vision way to better eyesight is the most innovative and effective self-help approach ever. Its key element is the simple and easily mastered technique of self- hypnosis. Hypno- Vision will help improve your eyesight quickly, with long-lasting results.

HYPNOSIS AND ACCELERATED LEARNING By Pierre Clement,
Soft Cover.135pp - $12.95
A do-it-yourself tool for self-hypnosis, divided into three parts. 1) Getting acquainted with hypnosis; 2) Acquiring self-hypnosis; 3) Utilizing self-hypnosis as a powerful learning method, including strengthening of will power concentration and speed of reading.

Use Your Credit Card and Call 800-894-9766 – Visa, MC, AE
700 South Central Avenue, Glendale, CA 91204
www.WestwoodPublishingCo.com

FINANCIAL SUCCESS through CREATIVE MIND POWER
Originally Titled -The Science of Getting Rich
By Wallace D. Wattles Soft Cover-92pp Includes Cassette Tape #104 - $17.95
This small book is a practical manual intended for those whose most pressing need is for money; wish to get rich first and philosophize after. It has been responsible for the successes of thousands of Mind Power students in the half-century since it was first published.

SEXUAL JOY Through SELF HYPNOSIS
By Dr. Daniel I. Araoz & Dr. Robert T. Bleck - Soft Cover 222pp - $19.95
This remarkable book teaches you how to overcome sexual problems that can arise through no fault of your own. Through self -hypnosis you will learn to focus your thoughts and end the power of the past to inhibit the pleasure of the present. You will be able to overcome premature ejaculation and failure to reach orgasm. You will learn to increase the intensity of your sexual experiences and achieve a more complete fulfillment. You will also gain an understanding of how your past experiences may have been affecting the expression of your sexuality. INCLUDES AUDIO CASSETTE #115 Sexual Enrichment for Men OR #116 Sexual Enrichment for Women.

TRANSFORMING THERAPY A New Approach to Hypnotherapy
By Gil Boyne Hard Cover.416 pp - $37.50
Here is a radically different approach to people helping. Boyne has created a unique system that speaks simply yet eloquently to the issues of filling our deepest needs and realizing our highest potentials. Boyne focuses on solving problems by stimulating the inner creative mind. Includes techniques, and complete verbatim transcripts of live therapies. This book brilliantly illustrates how Boyne's methods are currently redefining the meaning and essence of hypnotherapy.
"This book is a vivid, dramatic, clinical view into the innermost recesses of clients' emotional lives. Boyne is a gifted and creative therapist who has created a highly effective approach to hypnotherapy. "
Robert F. Reid, III, Ph.D., Professor California State University, Northridge

FREE CASSETTE WITH YOUR PURCHASE OF **TRANSFORMING THERAPY**
"Success Programming for the Hypnotherapist"
The only motivational program created exclusively for the hypnotherapist. It instills powerful confidence in the ability to use hypnosis creatively and to build and maintain a successful practice.

HYPNOSIS AND THE LAW   By Dr. Bradley Kuhns - Hard Cover.219 pp - $20.00
This training manual in forensic/investigative hypnosis is an exciting addition to the literature on hypnosis. Includes proven methods for dramatically improving recall, recollection enhancement and memory refreshment of victims and witnesses; plus transcripts of hypnotic sessions in major criminal cases.

HYPNOTISM AND MYSTICISM OF INDIA
By Ormond McGill - Hard Cover, Illustrated.203pp - $22.50
Noted author and hypnotist McGill reveals how the real mysticism and magic of India is accomplished. His detailed instructions for developing the powers of Oriental hypnotism are drawn from the secret teachings of the Masters of India, where he lived and studied for several years.

THE HEALING POWER OF FAITH: A Study of Alternative Treatment Modalities
By Will Oursler Soft Cover.366pp - $12.95
Throughout America, groups of people are meeting for the purpose of initiating healing. Some seek healing in churches and prayer meetings, while others take classes to learn spiritual healing methods. Adherents of spiritual healing have very different ideas of what illness and healing really are. Spiritual Healing systems stand in contrast to traditional medicine and challenge it, and the new kinds of thinking they promote are symptoms of profound changes in our society and in ourselves.

Use Your Credit Card and Call 800-894-9766 – Visa, MC, AE
700 South Central Avenue, Glendale, CA 91204
www.WestwoodPublishingCo.com

ANALYTICAL HYPNOTHERAPY By E.A. Barnett. M.D. Hard Cover 495pp - $32.50
A unique blend of analytic and direct suggestion techniques. Clearly written so that they may be understood by both hypnotherapist and layperson alike. The book is well researched and very effective in its explanation of practice. A section on case histories forms a major part of the work.

THE MIRACLE OF MIND POWER By Dan Custer Soft Cover.263pp - $12.95
A stimulating and inspirational volume full of answers as to how and why people grow, Custer's classic book demonstrates the potential for better health, greater happiness, and increased prosperity through the dynamic power of the mind.

BEYOND WORDS By Paula Slater& Barbara Sinor Soft Cover-271pp - $12.95
When we attempt to describe our inner knowledge, words seem inadequate since the fullest understanding is always "beyond words." Beyond Words is a brief encyclopedia of articles on more than 120 topics with a list of reference books at the end of each topic   Topics include "Metaphysics", "Altered States of Consciousness", "Transformation", and "New Age".

THE NEW ENCYCLOPEDIA OF STAGE HYPNOTISM
By Ormond McGill Hard Cover- 605pp - $64.95
The most comprehensive work ever produced on stage hypnotism. How to design, develop and perform a modern hypnotic show. Over a hundred different methods of hypnotic induction are described in detail. Includes openings, routines, advertising, business and legal aspect. The language is clear and simple. The approach is practical and down-to-earth.

"CRAZY" THERAPIES
 By Margaret Thaler Ph.D. & Janja Laich - Hard Cover.263pp   - $23.00
An expose' of many of the strange and esoteric alternative therapies that flourish at this time, often combined with "hypnotherapy." This is a guide that exposes the truth about offbeat therapies and some individuals who call themselves a hypnotherapist. It includes a variety of case histories of people who have experienced controversial therapies and also distinguishes between what is good and legal and what is not.

How to Help Yourself and Those You Love STOP SMOKING
By Jim Liles, M.S.W.Soft Cover-44pp + 2 Tapes - $19.95
This highly effective system does not depend on will power. The urge to smoke is eliminated without anxiety, withdrawal, or weight gain. Written to assist therapists and smokers in curing the smoking habit. The techniques of hypnosis are explained so that the smoker can examine their behavior, understand it, and mentally prepare to change it. Practical and enlightening. Should be read by anyone wanting to stop smoking or seeking to help someone else. Cassettes included – Stop Smoking Today and Appetite Control.

HYPNOTISM TRAINING COURSE #101 By Gil Boyne
Eight audio tapes in a binder plus a 98-page manual with numerous scripts. - $99.95
Fifty hours of classroom training edited down to eight hours of vital material. You'll hear students being hypnotized, Boyne's answers to students' questions, all major lectures, principles, techniques, and methods.

8 BEST SELLING SELF-HYPNOSIS CASSETTES
By Gil Boyne 8 audiotapes in a binder & 36pp manual - $99.00
The eight best selling audio tapes and a manual for creating your own power programming cassettes as well as the complete word-for-word scripts of the included tapes. Topics include self-confidence, concentration & memory, success, weight control, verbal skills, self-discovery, and health and stop smoking. A wealth of information.

MARKETING SELF-HYPNOSIS & Other Group Programs By Gil Boyne 99pp-8.5x11 - $35.00
Learn the techniques and attitudes for your success in preparing and marketing group programs. Includes, how to create you brochure, where to hold your class, selling a self-hypnosis course, marketing books and tapes and television interviews. All the information you need to create a successful, income-generating program.

HOW TO TEACH SELF-HYPNOSIS By Gil Boyne 186pp-8.5x11 - $35.00
A complete word-for-word transcript of an actual weekend self-hypnosis course given at a local college. All the necessary lessons and demonstrations you will need for a successful and inspiring self-hypnosis course.

Use Your Credit Card and Call 800-894-9766 – Visa, MC, AE
700 South Central Avenue, Glendale, CA 91204
www.WestwoodPublishingCo.com

TRAINING VIDEOS
All Videos Available in NTSC or PAL

STAGE HYPNOSIS

PART ONE: GIL BOYNE – From 1960 to 1965, Gil Boyne entertained thousands with his "Hilarious Hypnosis" Stage Show in nightclubs throughout the USA This video tape combines one full hour of highly-skilled stage hypnosis techniques with the hilarious antics of a stage full of subjects.

PART TWO: ORMOND MCGILL -, Dean of American Hypnotists, presents a fascinating and mirth provoking one-hour show in his unique style. This is your opportunity to compare and learn from the art of two of the world's great stage hypnotists. *2 hours • $75.00*

HYPNOTIZING DIFFICULT SUBJECTS
OVERCOMING "I CAN'T BE HYPNOTIZED"

PART ONE: DAMIEN (MISUNDERSTANDS TRANCE) -- A 22-year-old male college student has had seven sessions with two different hypnotherapists and reports he has never "been in a trance." Intake interview, instant standing induction, eye catalepsy, arm catalepsy, arm levitation, heavy left arm, handclasp response plus self-hypnosis training session. In posthypnotic interview, Damien reports he is convinced he was in a trance.

PART TWO: BOB (FEAR OF FAILURE) -- Bob, a 72-year-old Hypnotherapist, has been unable to experience trance in spite of his many efforts to do so. Using age regression, Boyne uncovers mother's early script: "You'll never amount to anything". Bob enters into a deep trance complete with several tests. Boyne then teaches him self-hypnosis and he comes up from the trance amazed and radiant. *1 hour, 33 minutes • $75.00*

INSTANTANEOUS INDUCTIONS
(STANDING)

PART ONE: TWO SUBJECTS – Total Loss of Equilibrium · Eye Catalepsy · Arm Catalepsy · Deepening by Compounding · Non-Verbal Reinduction · Waking Hypnosis Creating Partial Amnesia · Creating Total Posthypnotic Amnesia · Induced Speech Inhibition · Second Instantaneous Induction · Eye Catalepsy Test · Rule of Reverse Mental Effort · Teaching Self-Hypnosis to Subject · Healing Suggestions.

PART TWO: COLIN -- A student from England has never been hypnotized before. Gil Boyne demonstrates Instantaneous Induction (standing) · Deepening by Disorientation · Deepening by Realization · Rule of Reverse Mental Effort · Deepening by Rocking Subject · Arm Catalepsy · Automatic Motion · Deepening by Pyramiding · Handclasp Response · Creating Somnambulism · Creating Posthypnotic Proof-of-Trance · Conditioning for Posthypnotic Reinduction by Repeated Instant Inductions · Posthypnotic Talk · Posthypnotic Reinduction · Trance Termination.

PART THREE: MOLLY (SEATED INDUCTIONS) Includes: Hand Pressure Induction · Gazing-at-the-Moon Induction · Trance Termination · Arm Levitation (Eye Catalepsy and Heavy Left Arm) · Two-Finger Induction · Clearing the Mind · Reversed Handclasp Induction. *
*Fully Annotated ! *1 hr, 47 mins $75.00*

HYPNOTISM TRAINING FILM #501
Gil Boyne Teaching and Demonstrating

Hypnotherapist, Gil Boyne demonstrates five methods of Instantaneous Induction and simultaneously explains the processes in non-technical language as he works with ten subjects. Vivid examples of Testing and Deepening, Training the Client, Developing Rapid Rapport and Re-Educating the Client using students in attendance. Includes Arm Levitation · Eye Catalepsy · Arm Catalepsy · Automatic Motion · Key-Word Reinduction · Ten Methods of Deepening the Trance Posthypnotic Suggestions · Amnesia and other hypnotic phenomena *1 hour, 45 minutes*

Special Offer - **Our best-selling video at a special price: $37.50! Includes a complete word-for-word transcript of the video absolutely *FREE!***

HYPNOTISM TRAINING FILM #300

PART ONE: ADVANCED HYPNOTIC TRAINING -- Actual live, unrehearsed demonstrations filmed in a classroom setting using the students in attendance. Gil Boyne teaches and demonstrates instantaneous inductions, testing and deepening, training the client, developing rapid rapport, and re-educating the client.

PART TWO: HOW TO VISUALIZE A frustrating problem for hypnotherapists is the number of clients who report they are unable to visualize or use visual imagery. Here is how you can finally overcome that problem— forever. At a training seminar, a student informs Gil Boyne that he is unable to visualize. Watch as Boyne hypnotizes the subject and creates a process in which the subject "sees, hears, tastes, feels and smells." *1 hour, 45 minutes • $49.95*

TRANSFORMING THERAPY:™
A NEW APPROACH TO HYPNOTHERAPY
by GIL BOYNE

LEE
The San Diego Stutterer

In a dramatic two-hour hypnotherapy session using age regression and "uncovering techniques" Gil Boyne unveils the "battered child" syndrome and fear of castration as an initial sensitizing event for a life-long pattern of stuttering. Three years later, Lee remains totally free of stuttering. Gestalt dialogues, bodywork techniques and Parts therapy. *1 hour, 33 minutes • $75.00*

BUNNY PHYSICAL PAIN FROM EARLY SEXUAL ABUSE

Boyne demonstrates instantaneous inductions with several subjects. While testing one of them by making her upraised arm rigid she exclaims, "It's a miracle!" She explains that she has been unable to lift her arm higher than her shoulder for over two years. In an exciting and highly dramatic age regression Boyne discovers the cause of her arm, neck, and shoulder problems to be a result of early sexual abuse by her alcoholic father. Using several original and unorthodox techniques, Boyne creates a complete release from these disabling symptoms. Includes one-year follow-up. *1 hour, 22 minutes • $75.00*

TED
LAW STUDENT EXAM ANXIETY

Ted is a highly-intelligent young married man, who is about to take his final exam to graduate from law school. The exam is critical because if he flunks he cannot continue his studies at the school. Intake interview fails to reveal any indications of subconscious "scripts" at work. Gil Boyne's Power Programming is used as well as self-hypnosis instruction and the daily use of hypnosis tape at home is prescribed. In a follow-up session Ted reports his amazement at his calm and efficient behavior during the exam and his almost total recall. Further programming to prepare Ted for the Calif. bar examination. Follow-up report shows Ted reporting his successful passage of the bar exam. *2 hours, 18 minutes • $95.00*

FEAR OF CRITICISM & CURSE OF PERFECTIONISM

Gil Boyne's lecturing teaches the crippling effects of the fear of criticism and curse of perfectionism. He works with two subjects (Miriam and Sam); and discovers "childhood scripts" including the compulsive people-pleaser who "Won't say no." *53 minutes $49.95*

MARY - THE CHRISTMAS TREE ANGEL AND THE DEVIL

Mary learned as a child that it's "nasty" to feel good. Regression uncovers the discovery of "good feelings" in the genitals. Mother warns Mary, "Nice girls don't do that." As an adult, Mary avoids sexuality through obesity and an unattractive appearance. A two-day follow-up shows Mary nicely dressed, with her hair styled and groomed. She reports a different body image and new eating patterns. *1 hour, 6 minutes · $75.00*

BUD - Born to Lose

A depressed male in his mid-fifties is convinced that he is a loser in life. Suffers from alcoholism, insomnia, low self-esteem, self-isolation and negative thinking. In two one-hour sessions on consecutive days, Bud experiences an amazing personal transformation. Filmed live before a hypnotherapy class of forty-five therapists in Chicago. Shows age regression, abreaction, Gestalt dialogues and many of Gil Boyne's original uncovering, reprogramming techniques. *2 hours • $75.00*

HOLLY/PAT
PART ONE: HOLLY ("YOU SCARE ME")

A young woman in her mid-twenties breaks into tears in the first day of a Clinical Hypnotherapy course. When instructor Gil Boyne questions her she says, "You're scaring me." This seems a paradox since Boyne has not spoken directly to her in the class. He suggests that he hypnotize her to discover the background of her emotional upheaval. In minutes she is regressed to a terrifying scene with a threatening stepfather. Abreaction, re-education, rescripting and closure occur in rapid succession and the projected fear of an animated authority figure is dissipated.

PART TWO: PAT (FEAR OF PUBLIC SPEAKING)

A mature, intelligent female hypnotherapy student reports a fear of public speaking. She states that she "always sounds haughty" when speaking to a group. A comprehensive intake interview fails to reveal any evidence of negative childhood experiences or identifications. Trance is induced and deepened and a highly specialized program of affirmations and visualizations is presented. *46 minutes • $75.00*

APRIL
SEXUAL ABUSE

A student develops anxiety viewing case histories. Session begins with Gestalt dream work then age regression reveals sexual abuse. April developed belief that her genitals were "dirty" and this idea developed into a recurring theme that she was bad and "dirty." April contacts her repressed anger and rage and cathartic ventilation occurs. The use of Transforming Therapy™ techniques creates a willingness to begin a process of forgiving others and herself as well. This demonstrates that the sexual abuse client can recover self-esteem without having to physically or verbally assault the perpetrator. *55 minutes • $75.00*

KRISTEN - WEIGHT CONTROL AND CAREER MOTIVATION A 27-year-old former "Miss Los Angeles" complains of her inability to control her weight has greatly complicated her life and compromised her acting career. Boyne quickly identifies an intense fear of criticism and fear of rejection, and Kristen discovers how she uses her excess weight as a protective mechanism against her own sexuality and an avoidance of taking the necessary steps to enter into an acting career (i.e., "I can't begin as long as I'm overweight.").

In three sessions Boyne uses age regressions, Gestalt dialogues, "Saying Goodbye" and a unique form of suggestion programming. Kristen realizes the powerful subconscious impact of her mother's suggestions and her boyfriend's angry statement, "You'll have to sleep with many men to become a successful actress." As Kristen's perception of her emotion-driven behavior is changed, a new awareness of her personal responsibility in being overweight comes to her. She confidently states that she can now manage her weight, her family relationships and begin to pursue her acting career. *2 hours, 32 minutes • $95.00*

GIL BOYNE'S
HOW TO TEACH SELF-HYPNOSIS
HOW TO HYPNOTIZE YOURSELF AND OTHERS

Since 1956, Gil Boyne has taught self-hypnosis to more than 23,000 persons in Southern California. Boyne drew from his vast background of experience to create his most exciting project--a comprehensive course on "How To Teach Self-Hypnosis" consisting of seven hours of actual teaching on video cassette.

See and hear every element in the successful teaching of self-hypnosis, skillfully demonstrated in an actual class setting.

Includes a 99-page Marketing Manual and a complete word-for-word transcript of the seven-hour video cassette.
6 hours on 4 video tapes PLUS two manuals $195.00

Also available separately:
How to Teach Self-Hypnosis Transcript/Training Manual and *Marketing Manual*. $35.00 each **Save!** By buying both for $50.00.

Hypnosis for Healing and Pain Control This exciting video shows the use of the pain control method developed by Gil Boyne. Excerpts from three therapy sessions include: Cure of numerous warts on an eight-year-old girl • Cure of chronic migraine headaches in a 67-year-old woman • Controlling limb tremors in a client with Parkinson's Disease. *1 hours, 25 minutes • $35.00* **or FREE ! with minimum purchase of $300.00**

HYPNOSIS FOR MEDICAL EMERGENCIES
by Dr. Don Jacobs

USING SPONTANEOUS HYPNOSIS WITH THE SICK AND INJURED TO CONTROL PAIN & ENHANCE RECOVERY

Why is it that conversation at the scene of a medical emergency can have such a critical effect on the patient? This video shows that it is because frightened or seriously injured persons spontaneously enter into a hypnotic state of consciousness that makes them acutely responsive to certain kinds of direct or indirect suggestions.

Dramatizations and graphic illustrations present guidelines, strategies and techniques for gaining rapport and for giving suggestions and directives that can remarkably help patients control their own autonomic nervous system responses. These include: · Bleeding · Immune Response · Blood Pressure · Inflammation · Respiratory Functions · Heart Rate · Burn Injury Reaction · Dermatitis · Pain Response.

50 minutes • $75.00

THYROIDECTOMY SURGERY WITH HYPNOANESTHESIA
by Wm. S. Kroger, M.D.

A clinical professor at U.C.L.A. and author of *Clinical and Experimental Hypnosis*, Dr. Kroger demonstrates induction and deepening and creates glove anesthesia in a patient with thyroid disease.

In seven sessions, the patient is taught to create glove anesthesia and to transfer anesthesia to the neck. The fifth session is a rehearsal of the surgical operation and a explanation of each step to the patient.

In surgery, the patient hypnotizes herself and anesthetizes her neck and the operation is filmed and explained. Dr. Kroger creates total body catalepsy to minimize bleeding. Patient walks immediately after surgery.

16 minutes • $29.95

DERK
Self-Hypnosis and Ear Buzz

Student from Western Australia asked for help with a buzzing sound in his ears (tinnitus). Gil Boyne does a complete history and while Derk is in a trance, teaches him the use of "the control panel in the brain" to eliminate the buzzing. Teaches Derk self-hypnosis. After the session, Derk reports a great improvement in his control of the buzzing sound.

57 minutes • $75.00

ORIENTAL METHODS OF HYPNOTIZING
Ormond McGill

Based on his extensive travels in India, Ormond demonstrates the Oriental Method of Hypnotizing as you learn the power of visualization, affirmation and projection. Ormond's book *Hypnotism and Mysticism of India* has been a best-seller for ten years.

39 minutes • $15.95

SUCCESS ATTITUDES FOR YOUR HYPNOTHERAPY BUSINESS
Catherine Dumas · Durham, NC

Includes marketing, keeping costs down and quality up, ethics, the importance of continuing training, long-term reputation building, and short-term client flow. Created especially for the beginning Hypnotherapist, or the part-time Hypnotherapist who wants to become full-time. Catherine began her practice in North Carolina in 1992 and built to 20 clients per week in four months.

55 minutes • $15.95

TITLE	Quantity	Total

Westwood Publishing

FOR FASTEST SERVICE
Use your credit card and order by phone @ 818-242-1159 or E-mail to hypnotismla @earthlink.net

SHIPPING & HANDLING
Order Total
Up to $25.00 Add - $4.75
$25.01 to $60.00 Add $6.50
$60.01 to $125.00 Add $8.75
Over $125.00 **FREE!**
Foreign orders contact us for Quote

Subtotal	
Sales Tax **CA residence only add 8.25%**	
Shipping – see chart	
Total	

Your Name_____
Company Name_____
Address_____
City_____State_____Zip_____
Phone _____
Method of Payment
☐ Check Payable to Westwood Pub. ☐ Am. Express ☐ MasterCard ☐ Visa

Credit Card No._____
Expiration Date_____

700 S. Central Ave., Glendale, CA 91204 (818)242-1159
www.westwoodpublishingco.com